Children with Tracheostomies

RESOURCE GUIDE

SINGULAR RESOURCE GUIDE SERIES

Children with Tracheostomies

RESOURCE GUIDE

Marilyn K. Kertoy, Ph.D.
University of Western Ontario
London, Ontario Canada

SINGULAR
THOMSON LEARNING™

Australia Canada Mexico Singapore Spain United Kingdom United States

SINGULAR

THOMSON LEARNING

NOTICE TO THE READER

Publisher does not warrent or guarantee any of the products described herein or perform any independent analysis in connection with any of the product information contained herein. Publisher does not assume, and expressly disclaims, any obligation to obtain and include information other than that provided to it by the manufacturer.

The reader is expressly warned to consider and adopt all safety procedures that might be indicated by the activities herein and to avoid all potential hazards. By following the instructions contained herein, the reader willingly assumes all risks in connection with such instructions.

The Publisher makes no representation or warranties of any kind, including but not limited to, the warranties of fitness for particular purpose or merchantability, nor are such representations implied with respect to the material set forth herein, and the publisher takes no responsibility with respect to such material. The publisher shall not be liable for any special, consequential, or exemplary damages resulting, in whole or part, from the readers' use of, or reliance upon, this material.

Singular Staff:

HealthCare Publishing Director:
William Brottmiller

Acquisitions Editor:
Candice Janco

Editorial Assistant:
Maria D'Angelico

Executive Marketing Manager:
Dawn Gerrain

Channel Manager:
Jennifer McAvey

Project Editor:
Mary Ellen Cox

Production Coordinator:
Catherine Ciardullo

Art/Design Coordinator:
Connie Lundberg-Watkins

Printed in Canada

1 2 3 4 5 6 7 8 9 10 XXX 06 05 04 03 02 01

For more information, contact Singular Publishing Group, 3 Columbia Circle, Albany, NY 12212-5015; or find us on the World Wide Web at *http://www.singpub.com*

Library of Congress Cataloging-in-Publication Data
Kertoy, Marilyn.
Children with tracheostomies resource guide / Marilyn Kertoy.
p. cm. — (Singular resource guide series)
Includes bibliographical references and index.
ISBN 0-7693-0157-6 (alk. paper)
1. Tracheotomy—Patients. 2. Pediatric otolaryngology. 3. Physically handicapped children. 4. Trachea—Surgery. I. Title. II. Series.

RF517 .K474 2001
617.5'33'0083—dc21
2001047701

CONTENTS

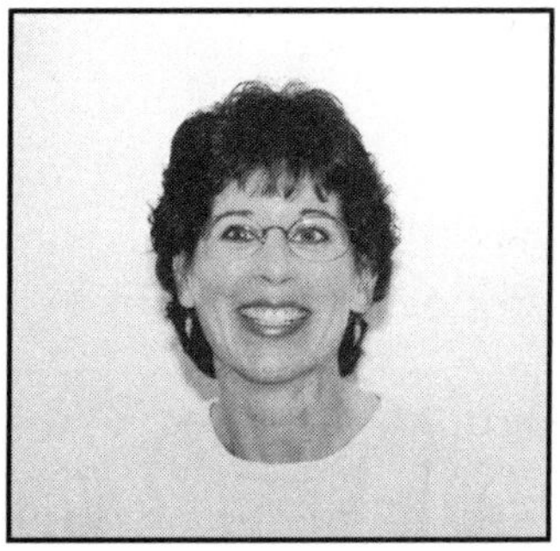

ABOUT THE AUTHOR

Marilyn K. Kertoy, Ph.D., CCC-Speech, Reg. CASLPO, is an Associate Professor in the School of Communication Sciences and Disorders, Faculty of Health Sciences, at the University of Western Ontario, London, Ontario, Canada. Dr. Kertoy's teaching and research focuses on the early development of infants and young children who are at risk for language delays, including children with long-term tracheostomies. She has conducted research and clinical work with children who are tracheostomized and their families for the past ten years.

Dr. Kertoy is also an Associate Researcher at the CanChild Center for Childhood Disability Research, McMaster University, Hamilton, Ontario, where she and her colleagues are studying participation in formal and informal activities by children and adolescents with physical disabilities. Dr. Kertoy is a member of a community-university research alliance investigating the factors and attitudes affecting the performance of children with special needs at school and in the community. These projects afford her the opportunity to pursue interests in the impact of cognitive, social and environmental factors on the development of language, and to work as a member of several interdisciplinary teams.

FOREWORD

The emblem for this series is a stylized road map. This symbol is intended to represent the goal of the series: to create books that serve as road maps to the care of communicative disorders. Like good road maps, each book gives the clinician an honest depiction of the territory, shows the various routes, and allows you, the traveler, to select the route best suited for your particular type of journey. Each book's author is someone who knows the territory about which he or she is writing, both as a clinician and a researcher. The hope of all involved in this series is that you will find the books useful and readable. Good traveling!

Ken Bleile, Ph.D.

PREFACE

The likelihood of speech-language pathologists providing consultation and/or treatment of children with tracheostomies and their families is great. Yet speech-language pathologists may not be confident in their ability to serve this population (Manley, Frank & Melvin, 1999).

The American Speech-Language-Hearing Association (1993) in the ASHA Position Statement and Guidelines for the Use of Voice Prosthesis in Tracheostomized Persons With or Without Ventilation Dependence, noted the need for speech-language pathologists to gain knowledge and then remain current in their knowledge of and experience with individuals who use advanced technologies. This knowledge and experience will likely be gained largely through continuing education and on-the-job training, rather than through academic and clinical-fellowship-year experience.

The purpose of this book is to take an initial step in sharing knowledge about children with tracheostomies in order to help in the ongoing training of speech-language pathologists. The book focuses on basic background knowledge essential to treating children with tracheostomies, as well as speech and language assessment and intervention for children with tracheostomies. The information provided here is not a substitute for direct observation or for hands on experiences with children with tracheostomies. Each professional will want to assess his/her comfort level and knowledge base and take additional steps to gain knowledge and experience in working competently with children with tracheostomies.

This book, like others in the Resource Guide Series, integrates research findings with clinical procedures. The characteristics of children with tracheostomies, the assessment procedures, and the intervention techniques were selected on the basis of the available research with children who have been tracheostomized. Because the research conducted with children with tracheostomies was sometimes limited, the author has borrowed assessment and intervention techniques that have been shown to be effective with other populations. These children included premature and low birth weight children in the intensive care unit, children with cerebral palsy, infants and toddlers at risk, and infants and toddlers with feeding and/or swallowing difficulties.

During the writing of this book, it became apparent that researchers and clinicians are at the start of their journey to generate and share knowledge about children with tracheostomies. Clinicians, researchers, and health administrators alike have a shared responsibility to promote knowledge and find ways to advance the sharing of knowledge about children with tracheostomies in order to better serve these children.

Clinicians are encouraged to present and publish procedures that are used effectively in everyday practice in bringing about changes in the speech and language of children with tracheostomies. Physicians and hospital administrators could join in pairing experienced and inexperienced professionals to promote hands-on experience in a supervised setting. Speech-language pathologists need graduated experiences, whereby they assume more responsibility as their skills increase so that the safety of the children is not placed in jeopardy. Health professionals can also share information from hospital databases about the numbers of children who undergo tracheostomies each year. Researchers may need to network to create larger databases to promote studies of speech and language characteristics and/or effective intervention procedures. Carefully designed single-subject studies to test intervention procedures would also be valuable to increase our current knowledge of effective interventions. By joining together on the path of knowledge gathering and sharing, we hope to overcome the current knowledge-practice gap, where approximately half of speech-language pathologists feel confident in working with individuals with tracheostomies.

ACKNOWLEDGEMENTS

Ellen Quart, who first introduced me to the complex issues faced by children with tracheostomies and their families.

Cindy Wheeler Ingham, for your clinical skills and research interests in children with complex medical histories.

The graduate students at the University of Western Ontario, who have contributed to research projects and shared a special interest in working with children with tracheostomies: Alison McVittie, Chris Guest, Rob Waters, Alison Morrison, and Gillian Bertleff.

Alison McVittie, who has been a friend and a supportive and knowledgeable colleague in working with children with tracheostomies the past 10 years.

The families who have shared their children, their time, and their homes to support research about speech and language development in children with tracheostomies.

Ken Bleile, who encouraged me to write this book.

Kathleen McGahan, who sorted, selected and typed the resources for the "Resources" section of this book.

Tanya Nermerich, who helped with proofreading and carefully prepared the index for the book.

Aunt Bertie and Uncle Paul, for a lifetime of love and support.

DEDICATION

Bud, Brock, Brice, Bevin, and Ashlee,

with gratitude for the health and happiness you

have enjoyed as children and young adults

and for the fun you bring to the Kertoy family.

SECTION

1

CORE KNOWLEDGE

WHAT IS TRACHEOTOMY?

Tracheotomy is a surgical incision that is made in the throat at the level of the second, third, and fourth tracheal rings during a tracheotomy operation. The surgical procedure creates a direct hole between the trachea and the skin that is called a tracheostomy. Throughout this book the term "tracheostomy" will be used and will refer to the resulting opening and tube placement. The opening or stoma is maintained by the insertion of a tracheal tube. The opening and tube placement occurs below the larynx and vocal cords. Prior to the surgery, the child's airway is maintained by placement of an endotracheal tube so that the child continues to receive air during surgery. Once the tracheal tube is in place, the child breathes directly through the stoma rather than through the nose and mouth. The tube is held in place by ties that go around the child's neck (Figure 1–1).

The tracheal tube usually fits tightly in the trachea so that maximum air pressure can be achieved. This tight fit inhibits the child's ability to vocalize. If the child can breathe adequately on his/her own, air goes from the stoma into the lungs and is exhaled again through the stoma. Some children have difficulty breathing on their own. If this is the case, a mechanical ventilator is connected to the tracheal tube to improve respiration.

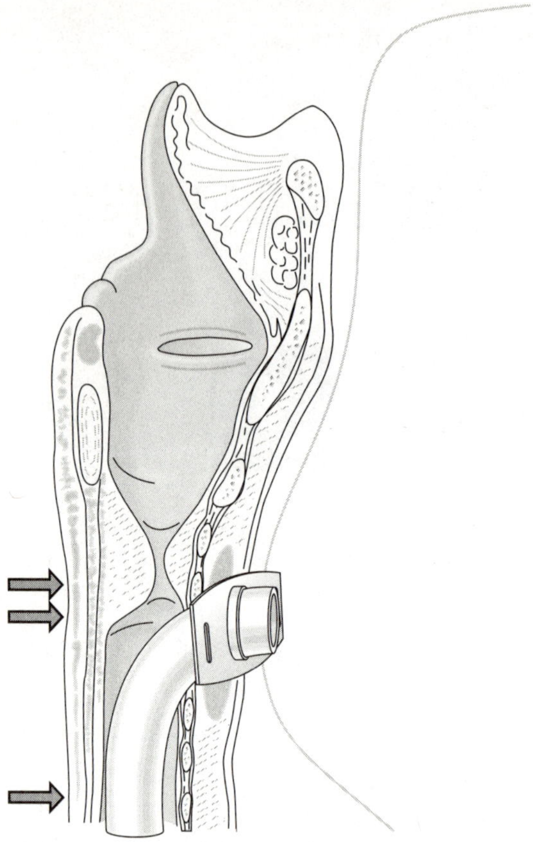

Figure 1–1 Tight-fitting tracheostomy tube (single arrow) or subglotic steriosis (double arrow) can impede the flow of air past the vocal cords and prevent vocalization. *Note.* From Simon, B. & Handler, S. (1981). The speech pathologist and management of children with tracheostomies. *Journal of Otolaryngology, 10*, pp. 440–448. Reprinted with permission of B. C. Decker, Inc.

PARTS FOR AND TYPES OF TRACHEAL TUBES

A tracheal tube has several parts: a tube, a hub, and a neck plate or flange. All tracheal tubes have an outer, slightly curved, cannula that goes from just inside the stoma, through the tracheal cartilage and down the trachea to just above the bronchi branch. At the proximal end of the tracheal tube (at the opening or stoma) rests a hub of 15 mm (15 mm is the standard outer diameter of most tracheal tubes). This hub is used to attach a speaking valve or an adapter for a ventilator, as needed. The third part of a tracheostomy is the neck plate. The plate sits behind the hub and rests against the child's neck. Some tracheostomies also have an inner cannula (Figure 1–2).

The type of tracheal tube placed in a given child will require a number of decisions. These decisions include: size of tube, length of tube, respiratory needs of the child, material tube is made of, use of inner and outer cannula or use of outer cannula alone. The child's age and weight are usually used as guides to selecting the size of a tracheal tube. The size refers to the diameter of the tracheal tube. Children who need high-pressure ventilation or frequent suctioning because of excessive secretions will require a tracheal tube that is larger in diameter than children without either of these needs.

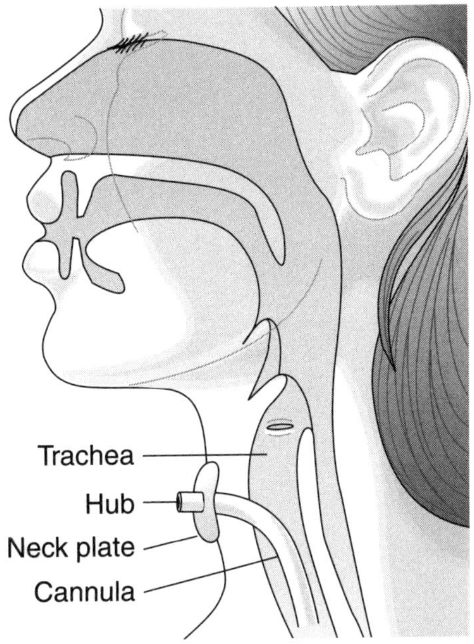

Figure 1–2 Display of outer tracheal tube, hub, and neck plate situated in a child.

The child's trachea is usually .55 cm in diameter, and ideally a tracheal tube will fill two-thirds of the tracheal space. For children with ventilator or suctioning needs, the tracheal tube should be fitted more tightly within the trachea, but allow for more space and better airflow within the tube itself. The length of the tracheal tube is generally long enough that the tube ends 1 cm above the carina (where the trachea branches into right and left bronchi) (Handler, 1993). A chest x-ray is taken to determine the appropriate length for each child. In very small children, the tracheal tube may need to be cut and custom fitted. Metal tracheal tubes are used less frequently in children than in adults. Children usually are fitted with either a polyvinylchloride or silicone tube because these materials are more pliable and less irritating than metal (Driver, 2000). Some tracheostomies have both an outer and an inner cannula. The advantage of a tracheostomy with an inner cannula is that it can be removed for cleaning. The disadvantage of an inner cannula within the outer cannula is that its use reduces the inner diameter of the tube and the amount of airflow.

Some tracheal tubes have cuffs. A cuff is attached to the tracheal tube and sits in the trachea along with the tracheal tube. When the cuff is inflated, a seal is created in the trachea, which permits air to flow in and out of the lungs through the tracheal tube, but not out the upper airway and mouth. The cuff is inflated by use of a pilot balloon outside the tracheal tube. The balloon is attached to the tracheal tube by a syringe. A child's cuff pressure is individualized and is measured with a manometer; the pressure is usually in the range of 20 to 25 mmHg. Overinflation of the cuff can cause unequal pressure against the tracheal and esophageal walls and result in tissue damage (Figure 1–3). Cuffed tracheostomy tubes are used infrequently in children because of the risk of damage to the developing trachea; thus they are used only when adequate ventilation cannot be achieved without a cuffed tracheostomy tube (Driver, 2000). Some children may have a cuffed tracheal tube right after the tracheostomy, but the cuff is usually not inflated. The cuffed tracheal tube is then changed to an uncuffed tracheal tube as the child nears discharge from the hospital.

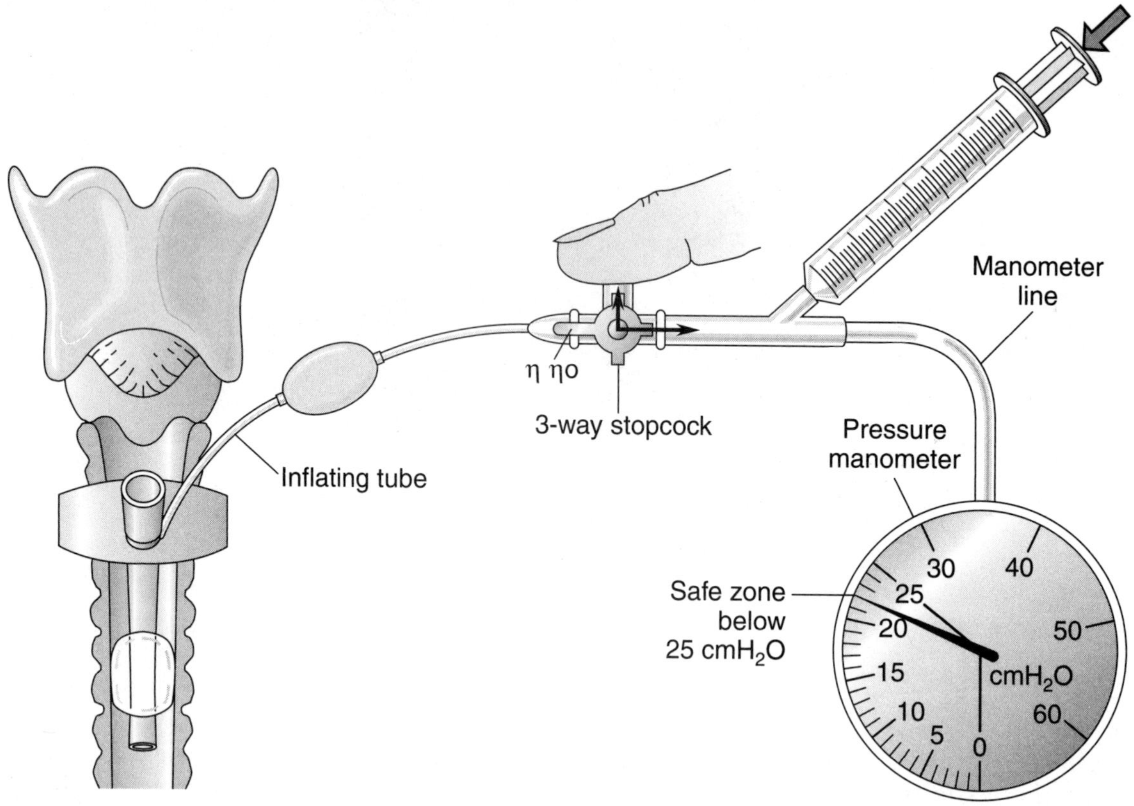

Figure 1–3 Display of tracheostomy tube with cuff, pilot inflating balloon, and pressure manometer. *Note.* From Kersten, L. D. (Ed.) (1989). *Comprehensive respiratory nursing: A decision making approach.* Toronto: W. B. Saunders Company. Reprinted with permission of W. B. Saunders Company.

It is important to understand the purpose of a cuff and its impact on the child's potential to voice and to swallow. Because air cannot be routed out through the upper airway and vocal folds when the cuff is inflated or if the cuff is too tight, the cuff must be deflated in order to achieve vocalization. The cuff also limits the elevation of the larynx during swallowing. Therefore, the cuff is deflated during feeding and swallowing. A special type of foam cuff (Bivonia Medical Technology, Inc.) is made to reinflate on its own (Figure 1–4). Children wearing a foam cuff are not candidates for a one-way speaking valve or for occlusion of the cannula for speaking. Other complications of cuffed tracheal tubes may include tracheal malacia, tracheal grannuloma, tracheal stenosis, esophageal obstruction, and swallowing difficulties.

WHY IS A TRACHEOTOMY PERFORMED?

Tracheotomy is performed when young children are unable to take in adequate air on their own or expend excessive energy to breathe or are unable to clear the airway of excess fluids. Tracheotomy occurs when there is an obstruction or collapsing of the airway, when muscular, neurological, or developmental conditions impede adequate

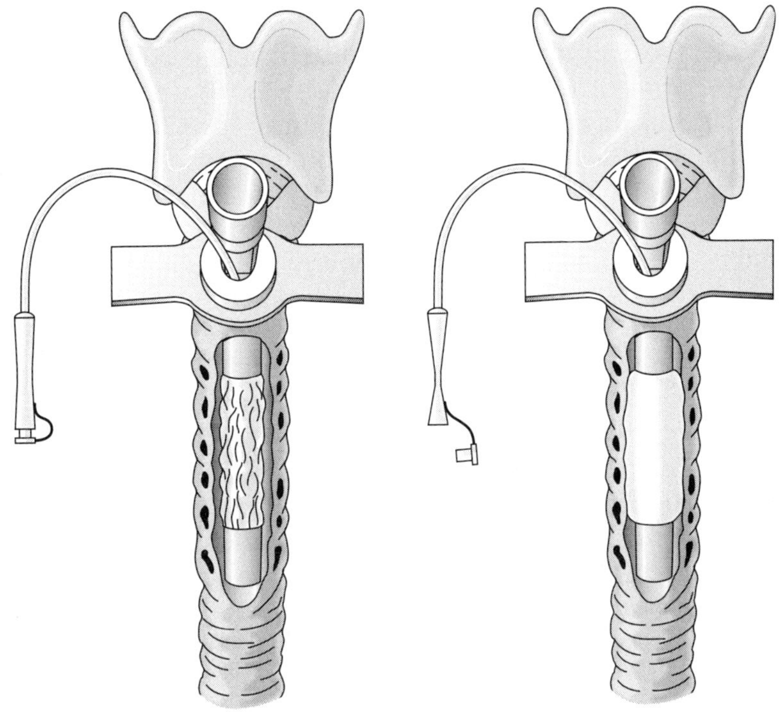

Figure 1–4 Display of foam-filled-cuff in the trachea in deflated and inflated positions. Reprinted with permission from Bivonia Medical Technologies, Gary, Indiana.

respiration, or when clearing of fluids from the airway does not occur via coughing or swallowing.

WHEN DOES TRACHEOTOMY OCCUR IN CHILDREN?

Many tracheotomies occur prior to the child's first birthday. Albamonte, Jerome, Diwadkar, & Seid (1993) reported that 85% of tracheotomies were performed in children under 1 year of age. Arvedson and Brodsky (1992) reported 60% of patients (37 of 62 patients) underwent tracheotomy prior to 18 months of age. Singer, Wood and Lambert (1985) reported that 45% of children in a sample of 100 had undergone tracheotomy prior to 13 months of age. The age at which tracheotomy occurs is important for speech, language, and feeding development. If the tracheotomy occurs prior to the child's first birthday, the tracheostomy is in place at a time when the child would normally have the opportunity to practice and hear their own vocalizations. Hearing one's own vocalizations appears to facilitate vocal development and language by serving as a "phonetic guidance system" (Locke & Pearson, 1992, pg. 110).

WHO IS THE CHILD WITH TRACHEOSTOMY?

As speech-language pathologists, we tend to focus on the impact of tracheostomy on speech and language in children who have undergone long-term tracheostomy, which is a tracheostomy that occurs prior to 13 months of age and is in place for 28 days or longer (Bleile, 1993). We think of the child with tracheostomy as a child who has undergone a surgical procedure that leaves him/her with an opening in the neck and unable to vocalize. While both of these observations are true, to be able to better understand the child with long-term tracheostomy, we need to recognize the larger population of children who were born prematurely or who have experienced various health conditions that necessitated the tracheostomy. The health condition that brought about the tracheostomy and the early environment of the child may have as great an impact on the child's long-term development as the tracheostomy itself. Singer, et al. (1985) noted that 47% of children with tracheostomy (21 of 45) experienced physical or neurological disease, while 21% (9 of 45) did not experience physical or neurological difficulties. In another study by the same researchers, 21% (33 of 130 children) survived, but experienced intellectual or neurological difficulties, while another 25% (32 of 130) of survivors had no intellectual or neurological problems. Children with tracheostomy might be divided into two broad categories with various health conditions that encompass those broad categories: the child born prematurely and/or of low birth weight, and the child with airway anomalies.

Premature, Low-Birth-Weight, and Small-for-Gestational-Age Children

Primary conditions associated with tracheostomy are prematurity (gestational age less than 37 weeks) and low birth weight (weighing less than 2500 grams). Premature children have a higher risk than full-term children for experiencing lung disease because the lungs have not had time to develop completely. Premature children are also at considerable risk for brain hemorrhage, because the central nervous system is not fully developed at birth (Goldson, 1996). In Canada, nearly 21,000 low-birth-weight infants (5.7 % of all births) were born each year from 1980 to 1990 (Levitt, Watters, Chance, Walker, & Avard, 1993). Children who are born prematurely are also likely to be low in birth weight. Singer, et al. (1985) reported that more than half of the 100 children they sampled with tracheostomy were born prematurely. One-third of the sample weighed less than 1500 grams at birth. Low birth weight is the factor most frequently associated with poor developmental outcome (ASHA, 1989).

Children can also be born at full gestational age and be small for their age (SGA; Gallagher & Watkin, 1998). These children show slow intrauterine growth patterns and are at or below the 10th percentile for size for gestational age. Approximately 20% of children who are small for gestational age experience small head circumference and are at risk for cognitive and central nervous system problems (Gallagher & Watkin, 1998). Singer, Kercsmar, Legris, Orlowski, Hill, and Doershuck (1989) reported slower growth rates in children with tracheostomy, but the slower growth patterns were not felt to be attributable directly to prematurity.

Low birth weight and prematurity may result in secondary conditions that place children at further risk for poor developmental outcomes. Children in respiratory distress frequently require mechanical ventilation in addition to tracheostomy. The tracheostomy creates an airway, and the ventilator presents a steady supply of oxygen to children who are unable to take in enough oxygen on their own. Thirty percent of formerly premature children compared to 5.6% of nonpremature children use technologies (ventilators, tracheostomy tubes, or gastrostomy tubes) (Slonim, Patel, Ruttiman, & Pollack, 2000). While mechanical ventilation is essential for sustaining oxygen intake, inaccurate monitoring of oxygen levels can lead to oxygen deprivation and serious consequences for the child's developmental progress (Bleile & Miller, 1994). Various health conditions associated with prematurity and low birth weight may require the long-term hospitalization of the child. During hospitalization, children do not have the normal supportive environment that they would experience at home. Neonatal intensive care units offer limited environmental stimuli for language development. Long-term hospitalization may also disrupt the normal parent-child bonds that form around feeding, bathing, and communication. This attachment is essential for the growth of early communication (Clarke-Stewart, 1973; Goldberg, 1977). Box 1–1 outlines the risks associated with prematurity, low birth weight, and/or poor growth rate.

BOX 1–1. Risks Associated with Prematurity, Low Birth Weight, or Poor Growth Rate

Intraventricular Hemorrhage
Respiratory Distress Syndrome/Bronchopulmonary Dysplasia
Mechanical Ventilation
Tracheostomy
Long-term Hospitalization
Cerebral Palsy
Developmental Delay

Airway Anomalies—Structural and Physiological

Some children who undergo tracheostomy do so because of congenital or acquired structural difficulties. Children may experience a number of structural conditions that restrict their ability to breathe. Table 1–1 outlines some of the major conditions that necessitate tracheostomy. These structural conditions may result in specific obstructions in the mandible, trachea, or vocal cords (i.e., congenitally small mandible, stenosis, or vocal fold paralysis).

Other airway anomalies can occur as the result of physiological conditions. These physiological conditions influence the motor control that children have to stimulate and/or control breathing. Spinal cord injury or central nervous system disorders may influence the level of control over stimulating and controlling breathing. Neuromuscular disorders such as Duchennes muscular dystrophy and cerebral palsy may also influence the child's ability to cough, to swallow, and to clear the airway of fluids (Colbert & Curran, 1991; Dormans & Pellegrino, 1998).

Mortality Rates in Children with Tracheostomies

Mortality rates in children who experience tracheostomy range from 2% to 28% (Wetmore, Marsh, Thompson & Tom, 1999). A survey of children with tracheostomy conducted in Germany showed a mortality rate of approximately 6% (19 of 280 cases) (Kleinsasser, Merkenschlager, Schroter, Mattick, Nicolai & Mantel, 1996). Deaths occur much more frequently from the underlying health condition(s) than from the airway obstruction or surgical procedure of tracheotomy. Some deaths do occur from airway obstruction, particularly after children are discharged from the hospital.

TABLE 1–1. Conditions that are Commonly Associated with Tracheostomy in Children

Conditions/Categories	Impact on Airway/Breathing
Obstructions in Tracheal/Laryngeal/ Epiglottal/Vocal Cord Area	
Stenosis	Narrowing of airway caused by trauma
Granulation of tissue	Build-up of tissue that leads to partial obstruction
Tracheomalacia	Laxity, floppiness of the structure
Vocal fold paralysis/incoordination	Airway may be obstructed
Congenitally small oral cavity or mandible (Pierre Robin, Treacher-Collins, Goldenhar, Haywell Syndromes)	Airway may be partially obstructed; small mandible may obstruct airflow; microagnathia, retroagnathia
Trauma	Damage to airway leads to obstruction, inability to take in air by mouth and nose
Lung Conditions	
Respiratory distress syndrome	Child unable to take in adequate oxygen
Bronchopulmonary dysplasia	Lung tissue damaged, child unable to take in adequate oxygen
Neuromuscular Disease	
Duchennes muscular dystrophy	Cough may be affected/inability to clear airway
Cerebral palsy	Increased incidence of respiratory disorders
Head and/or Spinal Cord Injury	
Spinal cord injury at neck level	Respiration may be affected
Head injury	Cough and swallow may be affected
Central Nervous System Damage	
Congenital central hypoventricular syndrome	Inability to stimulate breathing during sleep

Number of Children Affected in the United States and Canada

Bleile (1993) reported that the number of children who receive a tracheostomy ranges from 884 to 2,600 annually in the U.S. The number of technology-dependent children in the U.S. ranged from 680 to 30,000 based on a 1987 U.S. Congressional Report (Office of Technology Assessment, 1987).

FOR HOW LONG ARE CHILDREN TRACHEOSTOMIZED?

The length of the tracheostomy will depend on the reason for its initial placement. A review of recent studies of children who have undergone tracheostomy suggested that the number of tracheostomies may be declining in recent years, but the length of the tracheostomy continues to be greater than 12 months for the majority of tracheostomized children (Arvedson & Brodsky, 1992). Wetmore, Marsh, Thompson, and Tom (1999) noted that the mean duration of tracheostomy for those children in their sample who had undergone tracheostomy between 1981 and 1992 was 2.13 years.

Children appear to gain phonological and language skills gradually once the tracheostomy is removed (Locke & Pearson, 1990; Bleile, Stark, & Silverman McGowan,

1993). The full impact of the tracheostomy on later speech and language development requires further study as it is not clear whether children always attain speech and language skills within the normal range for their age (Bleile, 1998). Phonological difficulties have been noted in children following tracheostomy (Hill & Singer, 1990; Kamen & Watson, 1991; Kertoy, Guest, Quart & Lieh-Lai, 1999). The length and timing of tracheostomy appears to influence the speech and language recovery rate. Children who were decannulated after the development of some manual or spoken language (ages at decannulation ranged from 12 to 47 months) did more poorly than those children who were aphonic from birth and functioning below a 9-month language level at the time of decannulation (ages at decannulation ranged from 8 to 26 months) (Simon, Fowler, & Handler, 1983). Those health factors that necessitated the trachesotomy along with a child's inability to vocalize influence speech and language outcomes.

WHAT IS MECHANICAL VENTILATION?

Mechanical ventilation is a process whereby equipment is used to supply air to the lungs when the child suffers from inadequate ventilation or hypoxia. Tracheotomy and ventilation are two separate processes. The tracheotomy operation results in the creation of an airway through which the air supply can pass. Ventilation is the delivery of the appropriate air supply as opposed to breathing on one's own. The use of ventilation may follow the tracheostomy and continue until the child's respiratory status can be evaluated and stabilized. Tracheostomy is commonly performed after initial intubation of the child because of respiratory distress (Shinkwin & Gibbin, 1996). The tracheal tube supports the tracheal walls, which frequently weaken from the intubation. This support is also needed if the child is to receive oxygen support for an extended period. Ventilation has the benefits of decreasing the work of breathing and improving the oxygenation to a level appropriate for each child (Kersten, 1989).

There are two types of mechanical ventilators: positive pressure and negative pressure ventilators. Positive pressure ventilators are frequently used both in the hospital and at home. In positive pressure ventilation, air is forced into the lungs to expand the lungs and the chest wall. When the air is stopped, the lungs and chest wall recoil and return the pressure within the lungs to its normal state. The amount of air delivered may be pressure-or volume-controlled as well as continuous or intermittent. In negative pressure ventilation, negative pressure is applied outside the chest, which causes air to be sucked into the chest and lungs on inspiration. The chest and lungs recoil naturally on expiration. This type of ventilation may be used with patients that have neuromuscular problems and experience mild respiratory failure.

The delivery of air by a mechanical ventilator is not coordinated with speech in the same manner as it is in the child who talks on expiration. The ventilator can be set to deliver a specific concentration of oxygen at a rate of so many breaths per minute and can be activated with or without the assistance of the child's own spontaneous breathing. Therefore, the synchrony of forced exhalation and speech is not the same as the self-coordination of talking on exhalation. Further, the child with tracheostomy doesn't take in or expel air through the mouth, but rather through the stoma. The amount of air that may escape around the cannula upward into the mouth is far less than that in normal exhalation and will sustain only weak speech.

Although mechanical ventilation is essential for many children with lung disease, there are some disadvantages associated with mechanical ventilation. The child is at greater risk of infection, and oxygen toxicity may occur. Some children take long periods to wean themselves from the ventilation or fail to wean after long-term use (Mason & Watkins, 1992). Children who use ventilators are also at risk of respiratory failure if the tubes inadvertently become disconnected. Additionally, children are restricted in their mobility. Care needs to be taken so the child doesn't move beyond the length of the tubing and disconnect the ventilator.

Young children who use mechanical ventilators may be restricted in their ability to move about freely. The restricted ability to move may hinder the development of play as well as gross and fine motor skills. Children on respirators spend most of their time on their backs. Therefore, children have few opportunities to lay on their stomachs, lift their heads and bear weight on their arms and hands (Johnson-Martin, Jens, Attermeier, & Hacker, 1991). They also have few opportunities to flex their necks and trunks. These restrictions may hinder more advanced motor developments of creeping, crawling, sitting up and walking (Mason, 1993). Care needs to be taken to allow the child as much freedom in moving about as possible and to plan for motor activities that promote the normal sequence of gross motor skills. The speech pathologist and other professionals can encourage various motor skills from the supine position (child on back), but will also want to change the child's position to encourage a greater variety of motor skills (Box 1–2) (Johnson-Martin, Jens, Attermeier, & Hacker, 1991).

BOX 1–2. Major Motor Skills Children Learn in Supine and Prone Positions

Supine Position (child on back)
- Turning head
- Moving arms and legs
- Pulling hands to mouth
- Reaching for objects above or at side of body
- Pulling feet toward trunk
- Rolling from back to tummy

Prone Position (child on stomach)
- Lifting Head
- Supporting self on elbows, head up
- Extending trunk while supporting self on elbows
- Supporting self on hands, head up
- Reaching for objects with one hand while supporting self on one elbow
- Pulling forward on tummy
- Pivoting trunk
- Rolling from tummy to back

Note. From Johnson-Martin, N. M., Jens, K. G., Attermeier, S. M., and Hacker, B. J. (1991). *The Carolina curriculum for infants and toddlers with special needs*, pp. 36–37, Baltimore, Paul H. Brookes Publishing Co. Reprinted with permission of Brookes Publishing, Baltimore, MD, and the author.

WHAT ARE ONE-WAY SPEAKING VALVES?

A speaking valve is a one-way valve that fits on the hub of the tracheal tube (at the stoma). Air enters the stoma and goes into the lungs in the usual way with the valve in place. The stoma doesn't need to be occluded because the valve is designed to close on expiration, directing air from the lungs through the oral cavity.

The speaking valve requires that the external diameter of the tracheal tube be smaller than the tracheal lumen to ensure that the escaping air has an adequate airflow route. Children with a tightly fitting tracheal tube or children for whom the walls of the trachea have narrowed or collapsed around the tracheal tube do not have an adequate outward air route and are generally not good candidates for speaking valves. Children who have tracheostomies with cuffed tubes need to have the cuff deflated before the speaking valve can be operated and need to be able to tolerate cuff deflation. Children requiring a cuffed tracheal tube, whether with or without a ventilator, are usually not good candidates for speaking valves (Figure 1–5).

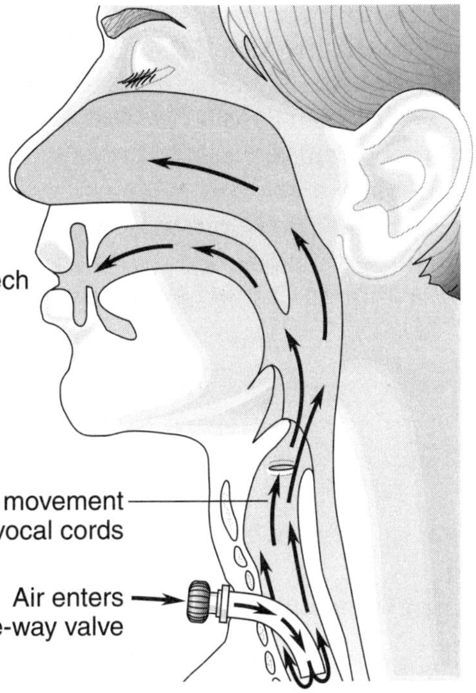

Figure 1–5 Display of airflow pattern through the trachea, larynx, and mouth with one-way speaking valve in place. *Note.* From Kersten, L. D. (Ed.) (1989). *Comprehensive respiratory nursing: A decision making approach.* Toronto: W. B. Saunders Company. Reprinted with permission from W. B. Saunders.

Children usually require an adjustment period to adapt to use of the speaking valve. A team of developmental pediatric specialists work together to develop a program for children with tracheostomies, including the evaluation of the feasibility of wearing a speaking valve. Ideally, a speaking valve is ordered by an ear, nose, and throat specialist (ENT) with the recommendations of the speech-language pathologist, respiratory therapist, pulmonologist, and family. A speech-language pathologist places the speaking valve on each child for the first time. The respiratory therapist is also present, along with a team comprising a respiratory therapist, an ENT nurse, and a pulmonologist. Children are frequently anxious at the first several fittings of their valve because they may have the sensation that they are not getting enough air. Children may be feeling the changes in air resistance when breathing in versus breathing out (sensation in oral, nasal, and pharyngeal areas). The child needs to adjust to the resistance of the air escaping through the oral cavity again. The speech-language pathologist (along with the respiratory therapist or nurse) generally assists with the child and family's ongoing adjustment to the use of the speaking valve, including fitting, removal, care, and trial placement for brief periods of time. Parents are taught how to easily twist the valve to remove it from the hub when the child becomes distressed. Team members answer questions for the family, demonstrate the proper use and cleaning of the valve, and help to reduce the family's fears. The speech-language pathologist works to have the child gradually tolerate the valve for longer periods. Once the child can tolerate the valve for 5 to 10 minutes at a time, the speech-language pathologist will initiate a program for the child to produce and increase audible vocalizations (Box 1–3).

BOX 1–3. Initial Placement of the Speaking Valve/ Working as a Team

- Obtain written or verbal permission from the otolaryngologist to place a valve.
- Prior to placement, an assessment of the child's physical, respiratory, and communication status should be completed by the nurse practitioner or clinical nurse specialist, pulmonologist or otolaryngologist, respiratory therapist and speech-language pathologist.
- The speech-language pathologist should complete a review of the child's chart to predict success (based on medical and airway conditions) and to rule out the presence of interfering factors.
- The respiratory therapist may suction the child prior to placement.
- The speech-language pathologist will occlude the stoma with a gloved finger to verify that the child can achieve airflow through the upper airway.
- The speech-language pathologist, respiratory therapist, and pulmonologist or otolaryngologist will be present at the initial placement of a speaking valve and will explain the physical procedure to the child and family.
- The family will also be informed of what will be done and what responses to look for in the child. They will be advised that the child will likely cry.
- The speech-language pathologist or respiratory therapist will physically place the speaking valve on the hub of the tracheostomy tube.
- If the child is on a ventilator, the respiratory therapist will disconnect and reconnect the appropriate tubing to accommodate the speaking valve.
- The speech-language pathologist will note whether there is airflow through the upper airway (breathing or crying by child).
- The child will wear the speaking valve briefly the first time (generally several brief attempts of several seconds, spaced several minutes apart, are completed).
- The respiratory therapist and speech-language pathologist will watch the child closely for signs of distress. The child's color, heart rate, excessive secretions, respiration and oxygen saturation are carefully monitored through physical responses and the output of the machines.
- At follow-up placements of the speaking valve, generally two professionals from the speech-language pathology, nursing, or respiratory therapy team are present to carefully monitor the child.
- The speech-language pathologist or respiratory therapist provides educational training and demonstrations for nursing staff and parents on the use of the speaking valve.
- The speech-language pathologist makes recommendations regarding the length of placement and number of times per day the speaking valve should be worn.
- Eventually, the nursing staff and parents assume the primary role in placement and removal of the valve, suctioning, and monitoring the child for signs of distress in the hospital and at home.

Note. Based on procedures recommended by Alison McVittie, speech-language pathologist on a pediatric critical care unit, London, Ontario. Printed with permission of the author.

Types of Speaking Valves Used with Children

There are several speaking valves commonly used for children. Four one-way valves are made to fit on the 15 mm hub of a tracheal tube: the Passy-Muir Tracheostomy Valve and Passy-Muir Ventilator Valve (Passy-Muir, Inc.), the Montgomery Tracheostomy Speaking Valve (Boston Medical Products), the Shiley Phonate Speaking Valve (Nellcor Puritan Bennett, Inc.), and the Hood Speaking Valve (Hood Laboratories). The Montgomery Tracheostomy Speaking Valve and the Shiley Phonate Speaking Valve come with cough release mechanisms to prevent the valve from coming off when the child coughs. The Passy-Muir Tracheostomy Valve, Montgomery Tracheostomy Speaking Valve, and Hood Speaking Valve come with models that fit onto ventilators as well. The Tucker Valve (Pilling Weck) is made to be used with the Jackson Sterling Silver Tracheostomy Tube and includes a hinged flap that opens on inhalation and closes on exhalation. The Passy-Muir Speaking Valve uses a biased closed procedure, which means that the valve is closed during rest. The valve opens on inhalation, but closes prior to the end of the expiration cycle. The closed bias feature is proposed to reduce secretions and permit ease of use for patients. (Figures 1–6 through 1–10 and "Resources").

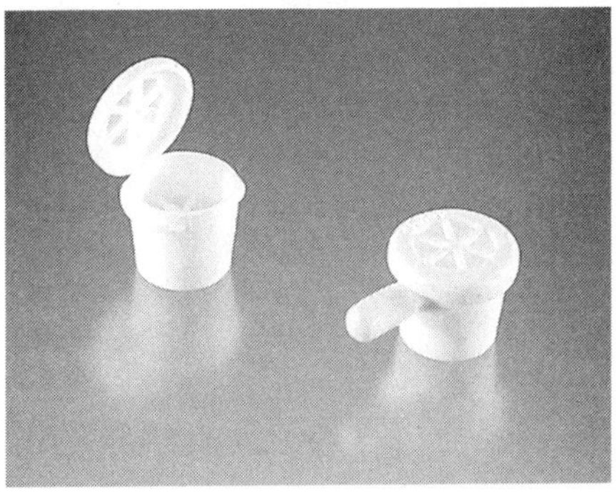

Figure 1–6 Shiley Phonate Speaking Valve. Courtesy of Nellcor Puritan Bennett, Pleasanton, CA.

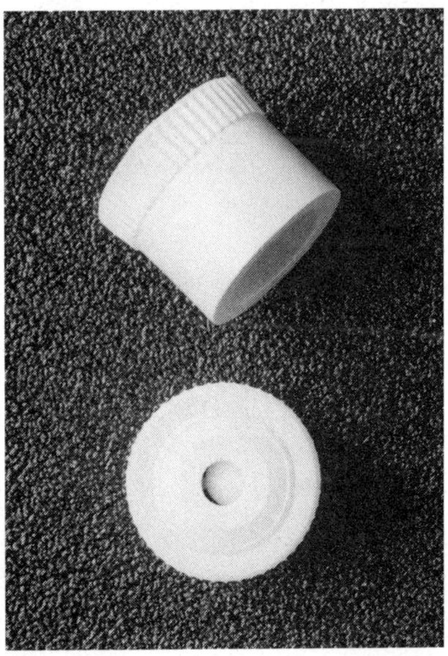

Figure 1–7a Hood Speaking Valve for Tracheostomy Tubes. Courtesy of Hood Laboratory, Pembroke, Massachusetts.

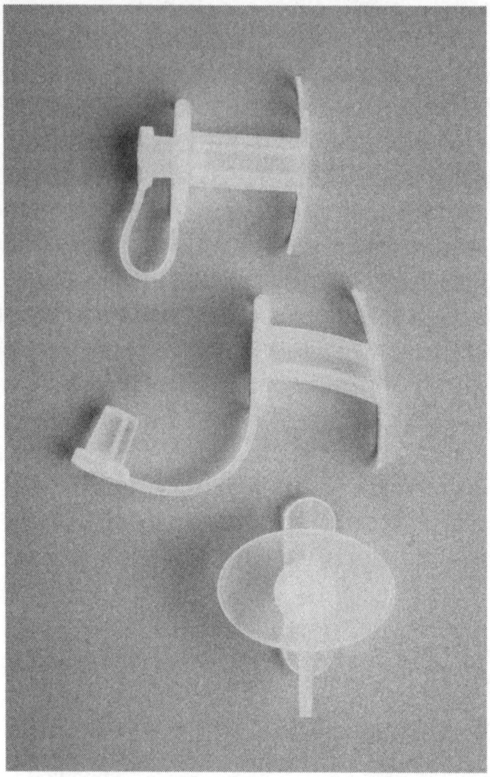

Figure 1–7b Hood Stoma Stents. Courtesy of Hood Laboratory, Pembroke, Massachusetts.

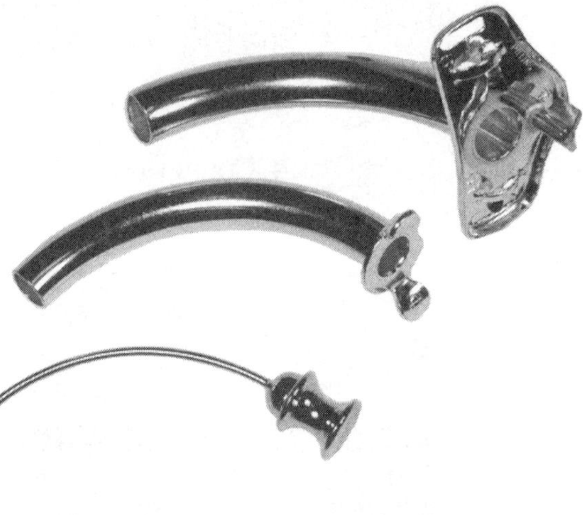

Figure 1–8 Tucker Valve with Tracheostomy Tube. Courtesy of Pilling Weck, Fort Washington, Pennsylvania.

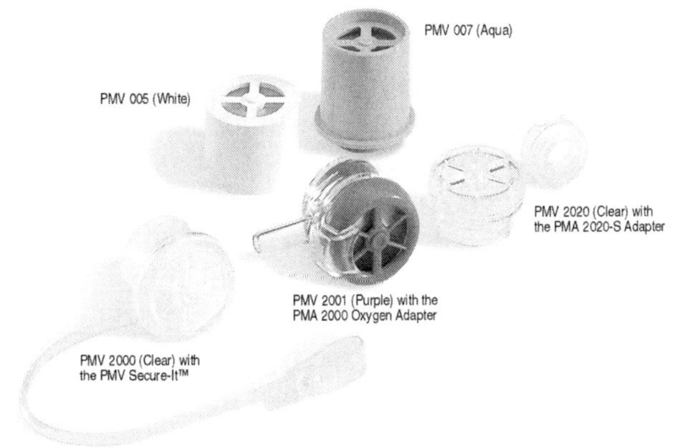

Figure 1–9 Passy-Muir Tracheostomy and Passy-Muir Ventilator Speaking Valves. Courtesy of Passy-Muir, Inc. Irvine, California.

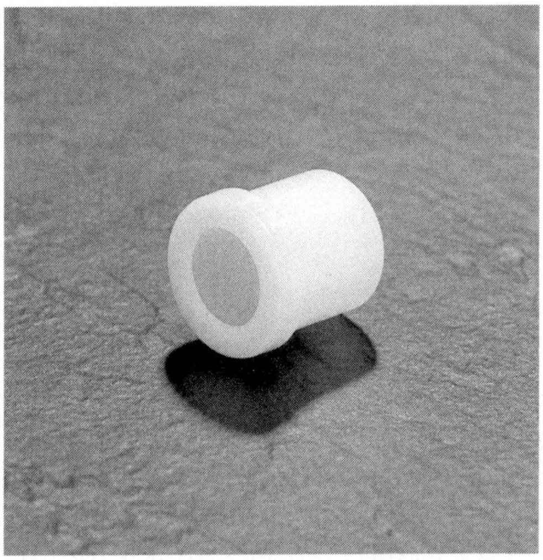

Figure 1–10 Montgomery Speaking Valve. Courtesy of Boston Medical Products, Westborough, Massachusetts.

WHAT IS DECANNULATION?

Decannulation is the medical removal of the tracheal tube on a permanent basis. The time at which a child is decannulated is dependent on two factors: (a) the child can breathe on his/her own without mechanical ventilation, and (b) there are no airway obstructions to hinder respiration (Handler, 1993). Both of these requirements are determined by the child's physician. The child is examined endoscopically to rule out potential airway obstructions. Possible obstructions can occur because of severe subglottal stenosis or laryngeal dysfunction. In extreme cases, surgery may be required to remove scarred tissue or to restructure the laryngeal and tracheal areas.

The actual decannulation procedure involves the removal of the cannula by a physician while the child is in the hospital. Decannulation is only performed after the child's independence in breathing has been established. After the tube is removed, the opening is covered with a bandage, and the child is observed to ensure adequate breathing for at least a day. The stoma will close on its own in many children. Sometimes tissue forms inside the stoma, and this must be removed surgically in order for the stoma to close completely. A build-up of epithelial tissue may occur when the child has been tracheostomized for a year or longer.

MODELS OF INTERVENTION AND THE IMPACT OF EARLY INTERVENTION

Care of infants who are premature and at-risk infants in a neonatal intensive care unit focuses on medical and developmental interventions. The need for environmentally and developmentally focused intervention became clear because many infants without significant neurological complications were still experiencing episodes of oxygen deprivation due to noisy intensive care environments and poor handling during routine care. Many intensive care units have adopted a model of developmental care based on the early work of Heidolise Als and colleagues to enact: (a) structuring of the environment, (b) timing and sequencing of care based on the child's readiness for care, and (c) continuous care from birth to discharge from the hospital (Als, Lawhon, Brown, Gibes, Duffy, McAnulty, & Blickman, 1986). By carefully observing the infant's behaviors using the checklist, Assessment of Preterm Infant's Behaviors, caregivers could time the care and interventions to fit the infant's readiness to adapt to the level of stimulation (Fitzgerald, Lester, & Yogman, 1982).

Many hospitals have developmental treatment teams in place to care for children who require intensive hospital care. Hospitals also vary in the level of care that is provided to infants who are at risk or experience severe, chronic illness. Infants may receive temporary care following birth for minor health problems from 12 to 24 hours postdelivery, or they may receive varying levels of specialized care in the intensive care unit over an extended period of time. Neonatal intensive care units (NICUs) are organized from Levels II to IV. Level II units provide care for infants with a medical crisis and increase in level of specialization and sophisticated technology to Level IV units, which provide highly specialized care for infants with complex medical conditions (Billeaud, 1998). In Canada, those children with the most critical health needs or who are ventilator dependent will receive care in neonatal intensive care, intensive care (ICU), or pediatric critical care units (PCC). Those children with less critical health needs and who are not ventilator dependent are treated in special care or ill infant nurseries.

The exact make-up of the developmental care team may vary from hospital to hospital. In the US and Canada, the neonatal intensive care teams generally comprise a neonatologist, neonatal nurses, a social worker, and a primary developmental specialist (Laadt-Bruno, Lilley, & Westby, 1993). These professionals serve as a core team serving the child and family and, in turn, collaborate with many other professionals in their specialties. For example, the social worker will help the family in locating support from community agencies. The neonatologist will confer with a team of medical specialists, depending on the child's specific medical concerns. The primary developmentalist may represent any of a number of professions (nurse, special educator, occupational therapist) and will be a primary contact for the family throughout their hospital stay, coordinate all services, and work with a team of rehabilitation and developmental specialists, including the speech-language pathologist.

The goals of the developmental care teams are to provide family-centered care, to provide consistent and continuous care to the child and family over a period of time, to plan and carry out a development plan for each child, and to provide the developmental care through team collaboration to achieve the best care for each child (Rossetti, 2001; Wyly, Allen, Pfalzer, & Wilson, 1996). The developmental programming includes modifications to the child's environment in the NICU and specific, individualized goals for each child regarding improvement in behavioral organization and self-regulation (See "Role of the Speech-Language Pathologist" in this chapter for further information).

Careful timing of medical care and developmental stimulation has resulted in shorter stays on respirators, greater gains in weight, and earlier success with bottle or breast feeding (Als, et al., 1986). Many infants (those weighing less than 2500 grams at birth) continue to be at higher risk for special education services based on a sample of 8,000 students aged 6 to 15 years in the U.S. (Chaikind & Corman, 1991). The findings from intervention studies generally suggest positive outcomes. However, the risk for developmental delays in children who undergo long-term hospitalization remains high, with rates as high as 50% of children experiencing developmental delays being reported (Goldson, 1996). Interpretation of the outcomes of intervention studies is also hampered by methodological issues and the use of controls who are not described and matched adequately (Meisels, Jones, & Stiefel, 1983). Better ways of describing the control groups are needed, with the inclusion of age and weight at gestation along with descriptions of the severity and chronicity of health conditions experienced by these children (Meisels, Plunkett, Pasick, Stiefel, & Roloff, 1987).

LONG-TERM VENTILATOR USE: ISSUES FOR FAMILIES

Some of the children who undergo long-term tracheostomy may also require ventilator assistance for long periods of time. Parents appear more satisfied and it is less costly when the child who is on a ventilator can be cared for at home. Strong case management of the child who is ventilator dependent appears essential to good treatment (Fields, Coble, Pollack, & Kaufman, 1991). Safety appears to be an issue, with higher mortality in the home than hospital setting. Families also report high levels of stress, which are related to caring for a child at home on a ventilator, and educational placements for these children are sometimes difficult to find.

Children with tracheostomies and/or mechanical ventilators being cared for in the home require effective case management, proper discharge planning and education of the family about their role in the medical care of the child with tracheostomy, and ongoing evaluation of the effectiveness of medical interventions in the home (Duncan, Howell, deLorimier, Adzick, & Harrison, 1992; Richardson, Student, O'Boyle, Smyth, & Wheeler, 1992; Willis, 1983). Parents of children with tracheostomies reported that maintaining a patent airway for their children, specifically the weekly changing of the tracheal tube caused most concern (Willis, 1983). Parents also expressed concerns about proper techniques for suctioning, humidification, and handling plugged tracheal tubes. In addition to concerns about maintaining a patent airway, parents of children with tracheostomies reported concerns about protecting their child from infection and concerns about the integrity of the skin near the stoma, along with concerns about speech and feeding development. These concerns highlight the need for educational programs and demonstrations about the care of the tracheostomy prior to the child's discharge from the hospital. Numerous researchers and hospitals have developed information and instruction programs or packages for families (see "Resources" and Web sites) (Barnes, 1992; Kennedy, Johnson, & Sturdevant, 1982; Rathlev & McNamara, 1982; Tippet, 2000).

ROLE OF THE SPEECH-LANGUAGE PATHOLOGIST

As discussed earlier, the child with tracheostomy may experience considerable risk for developmental delay, including speech and language delays. Because children who undergo tracheostomy are at risk for poor developmental outcomes, the speech-language pathologist, along with other professionals, will be involved in providing early intervention.The speech-language pathologist is likely to encounter children with tracheostomy on her/his caseload in several settings: hospital, home, preschool, and school. Table 1–2 outlines the settings and roles of the speech-language pathologist when working with children who have undergone tracheostomy.

TABLE 1–2. Work Settings and Roles of Speech-Language Pathologists Working with Children with Tracheostomies

Work Setting	***Roles***
Hospital	Involving families in communication with child
(Acute Care)	Answering family's questions about tracheostomy and expectations for their child
Home/Rehabilitation	Establishing a means of communication for the child
Hospital or Unit	Helping families establish developmental expectations for the child
	Helping families with care of tracheostomy and/or ventilator (may be done by nurse or respiratory therapist)
	Placement and care of speaking valve
Preschool	Improving communication for the child
	Facilitating transition of technology-dependent child to school
	Establishing and developing a means of communication
School	Improving communication for the child
	Facilitating inclusion and participation of the technology-dependent child at school
	Monitoring for the impact of long-term tracheostomy on speech and language

The role of the speech language pathologist serving children with tracheostomies in the hospital will vary according to the severity of the child's illness and the particular structure and policies of care for the hospital. The roles will also change as the child's health status becomes more stable. The speech-language pathologist will provide consultation to other professionals, to nursing staff, and to families, and will provide direct services to children regarding communication and oral-motor goals (Billeaud, 1998). The speech-language pathologist is likely to serve in a consultatory role while the child is in a Level III or Level IV intensive care unit (NICU in Canada). As the child's health improves and they move to the Level II nursery (ICU, PCC, or special care nursery in Canada), the speech-language pathologist will take a more direct service role. Because of the specialized care required of infants at risk and the specialized knowledge needed by the professionals who serve them, the speech-language pathologist will take on several important roles to serve the child and family best. Katz, Pokorni, and Long (1989) suggest that the speech-language pathologist is required to be an infant specialist, a consultant, a parent educator, and a program developer and advocate. The speech-language pathologist's job is not only understanding the preterm infant and knowing well the types of programming that he/she requires, but also being able to communicate the child's programs and needs to parents and other professionals in a clear and concise way. The effectiveness of the speech-language pathologist is dependent on his or her being able to work well with a team and to convince others about the importance of early communication programming.

Training and Knowledge Base of the Speech-Language Pathologist

The speech-language pathologist will perform many of the same assessment and intervention strategies that he/she would with other young or at-risk children under 3 years of age. For the speech-language pathologist who services medically fragile children in a hospital setting, the child with tracheostomy will be a regular caseload member. However, for the speech-language pathologist who is new to hospital or home settings or who works in the preschool/school setting, the child with tracheostomy presents particular challenges. The speech-language pathologist will want to familiarize himself/herself with a number of specialized areas and observe children with tracheostomy in a neonatal intensive care unit, local hospital, or feeding clinic (see Box 1–4) (Dunn, van Kleeck, & Rossetti, 1993a; Silverman McGowan, Bleile, Fus, & Barnas, 1993; VandenBerg, 1993).

The speech-language pathologist working in the hospital will also want to seek training in the use of several neonatal assessment tools (Als, Lester, Tronick, Brazelton, 1982; Brazelton, 1984). These measures assess the infant's responses to his/her environment and incorporate many developmental areas. In addition to increasing one's knowledge base, the speech-language pathologist will want to obtain direct observation of and experience with young children or adults who are tracheostomized (Manley, Frank, & Melvin, 1999).

A recent survey indicated that most speech-language pathologists have worked with at least one individual with a tracheostomy, but only half of the speech-language pathologists surveyed indicated that they were confident in servicing this population (Manley, et al. 1999). It is becoming increasingly apparent that speech-language pathologists will be faced with serving individuals who are tracheostomized (ASHA, 1993). It is also important that speech-language pathologists combine classroom knowledge with supervised, hands-on experience prior to undertaking the treatment of children who are tracheostomized. Supervised experiences may be obtained through job shadowing with other speech-language pathologists, respiratory therapists, or other professionals; or in settings with multiple speech-language pathologists, the new clinician might team with and be supervised by a speech-language pathologist experienced in working with tracheostomized patients. Medical settings may need to offer training programs for area speech-language pathologists in order that speech-language pathologists who serve children with tracheostomies will do so with the necessary knowledge and practical experience (Box 1–4).

BOX 1–4. Training and Knowledge Areas Important for the Professional Serving Children with Tracheostomy

- Cognitive, social, motor, and communication development of infants and toddlers who are developing normally or who are at risk
- Medical conditions associated with tracheostomy and medically fragile children
- NICU environment and the impact on early speech and language development
- Programs for developing a stimulating environment in the NICU
- Early prelinguistic signals and communication
- Strategies for involvement of parents in early communication
- Operation, toileting, and care of tracheostomy and mechanical ventilators
- Features and operation of speaking valves
- Physiology of respiration and impact of mechanical ventilation on respiration
- Impact of motor disorders on respiration and phonation
- Communication options for children with tracheostomy
- Feeding and swallowing issues for children with tracheostomy
- Supervised experience when working initially with children with tracheostomy

SECTION

2

COMMUNICATION ASSESSMENT FOR CHILDREN OF 0–3 YEARS WITH TRACHEOSTOMIES

NEED FOR ONGOING ASSESSMENT

The primary goals of communication assessment for a child with tracheostomy are to determine the child's current level of language, socioemotional, cognitive, and oral-motor skills and to establish an appropriate means of communication based on these skills. Children with tracheostomies represent a population with diverse developmental needs, based on the individual health histories and the health conditions which necessitated the tracheostomies. These children also experience fluctuations in health status that can affect communication, creating periods of little change or even regression in language milestones. Because the need for a means of communication remains critical throughout the period during which children are tracheostomized, it is essential that any and all communication opportunities and ways of communicating be evaluated on an ongoing basis. Children with tracheostomies should receive speech and language assessments frequently, and new communication options should be explored to match the child's changing communication status. By exploring how a child may be capable of communicating, the speech-language pathologist can establish, maintain, and modify an appropriate system of communication for the child and significant others. If each child has opportunities to communicate while tracheostomized, then the risks of long-term speech and language delays may be minimized. Because medical concerns of the child will occupy the attention of the family and other professionals, the speech-language pathologist may need to advocate for communication assessments and/or programming for each child (Box 2–1 provides assessment guidelines).

BOX 2–1. General Assessment Guidelines for Use with Children Who Are Tracheostomized

A. Assess multiple developmental areas in addition to speech and language because the child with tracheostomy may be at risk for delays in more than one developmental area.

B. Assess both receptive and expressive language. Just because considerable attention is paid to the child's expressive skills, don't overlook the development of receptive language. Receptive language skills should be in keeping with the child's nonverbal cognitive and play skills.

C. Match the assessment procedures to the situation. Many children with tracheostomies may start with fragile medical conditions that limit the assessment procedures that can be conducted. Begin with the use of observational checklists or parent report measures.

D. Move to standardized measures and to more in depth measures once the child's health status has improved.

E. The developmental needs of the child with tracheostomy will vary greatly, depending on the health condition(s) that brought about the tracheostomy. Some children with an airway obstruction that is corrected through use of the tracheostomy may present with near normal developmental profiles, while others with multiple health conditions and long-term respiratory distress may be at risk for severe delays. The speech-language pathologist should be ready for all possibilities.

F. Because of the complex histories of many children with tracheostomies, the speech-language pathologist is likely to conduct an assessment with other professionals or to seek the advice of/confer with other professionals to obtain a more complete picture of a child's functioning.

G. The speech-language pathologist will want to relate a given child's development to a normal developmental sequence, keeping in mind that many children with tracheostomies will proceed through a normal sequence, but at a much slower rate.

H. Assessment of the child with tracheostomy calls for constant reassessment to meet the needs of the child and family. The child's medical status may change rapidly (positively or negatively), and therefore the needs of the child and family will change.

GOALS AND CONTENT OF ASSESSMENT

This section provides assessment guidelines in the following areas: infant neurobehavioral organization, developmental screenings, cognition and play, social skills, oral-motor and feeding skills, gross motor skills, receptive and expressive language, and assessment of communication options. The content that is assessed will change as the child's health status and developmental needs change (Table 2–1). Several typical clinical situations that the speech-language pathologist may encounter and the goals of assessment in those situations are:

Situation 1: The child with tracheostomy who is in the Level III or IV intensive care unit and experiences severe health problems. The developmental age of children in this clinical situation may range from preterm to 4 months.

Goals: Assessment goals in this clinical situation will include the measurement of the child's neurobehavioral organization and responses to stimuli, the observation of oral motor skills, and the assessment of a child's early responses to the environment and the family's role in interacting with the child.

Situation 2: The child with tracheostomy whose health has stabilized, and who is gaining weight and has greater mobility and opportunities to communicate. This child may be in the Level II nursery or step down unit or may have been discharged to home a short time ago. The developmental age of the children may range from 4 to 12 months.

Goals: Assessment goals include measuring the child's developmental skills (language, social, motor, and cognitive) and observation of the child's means of communication. The speech-language pathologist may follow a general developmental screening with in-depth assessments of receptive language, play skills, and oral motor skills needed for speech. Efforts are taken to determine the child's ability to vocalize, to establish a means of communication, and to help the parents to interact with their child.

Situation 3: The child with tracheostomy who is likely to remain tracheostomized during the late prelinguistic and early linguistic period. Children representing this clinical situation may range from 8 to 24 months developmentally. Some of these children may remain in the hospital, but a larger proportion will be followed by speech-language pathologists and other professionals at home.

Goals: The assessment goals are to monitor the child's speech and language progress and the child's use of an effective communication system, and to identify areas of development that require stimulation to help alleviate long-term speech, language, and developmental delays.

Situation 4: The child who is recently decannulated, but who is gaining speech and language skills slowly.

Goals: Once the child is decannulated, the speech-language pathologist will continue to monitor speech and language development to ensure that the child continues to progress.

The speech-language pathologist may also see each of the scenarios in the same child as the child progresses, but continues to have a tracheostomy in place or to experience the aftermath of having a tracheal tube. The assessment procedures and guidelines reviewed here are not an exact or complete development sequence from 0–3 years, nor are they all inclusive. The guidelines were selected for their importance to this population or because of available information about application of the procedures to children who are at risk (Table 2–1).

TABLE 2–1. Goals and Content of Assessment

Child's Status	*Goals*	*Content Areas*
• Child has recently undergone tracheostomy and/or child's health is unstable	• Observe level of behavioral organization	• Infant Behavior Organization Assessments
	Assess signs of stability and stress	Behavior Checklist
Developmental level: preterm to 4 months	Parental observation of child's approach/avoidance behaviors	Checklist for observing child's responses to stimuli
	Assess child's oral-motor functioning and feeding	Oral-motor observation checklist/feeding assessments
• Child's health is stable	• Assess overall development (social, cognition, language)	• Infant developmental assessments Developmental sequence
Child is able to interact with environment	Assess receptive language	Receptive language measures/developmental sequence
Developmental level: 4 to 12 months	Assess play Establish parent-child interaction Assess means to communicate	Play measures Ability to vocalize
• Child's health is stable	• Observe development of communication	• Developmental sequences for vocalizations and gestures
Child is likely to be tracheostomized for several months or longer	Assess reasons to communicate	Development of communicative intents
Developmental level: 8 to 24 months	Encourage reciprocal interaction	Initiations, responses, maintenance of turns
	Establish communication system	See content below
	Assess areas needed to support various communication systems	Respiration Receptive Language Medical status Motor coordination Cognition Ability to vocalize
• Developmental level: 24 months and older	• Assess progress in cognition, phonology, receptive and expressive language	• Receptive language Expressive language Cognition Medical status
	Assess need for change in communication system on a regular basis	Note changes in content areas and modify system based on child's skills, needs

FORMAT FOR PRESENTING ASSESSMENT PROCEDURES

For each procedure reviewed in this section, answers to the following questions will be provided along with the research literature that supports the use of the procedure or provides information about the language performance of children utilizing the procedure.

Who? Indicates the age or health and developmental status of the child for whom the procedure is most appropriate.
What? Indicates the subject or topic of the procedure.
When? Indicates the circumstances under which the parent or speech-language pathologist might find using the procedure most helpful.
Where? Indicates the physical location or the functioning level of the child required to optimally complete the procedure.
How? Indicates the general instructions for completing the procedure. Specific instructions are frequently provided in a separate paragraph.
Why? Indicates the importance of the topic or procedure for children with tracheostomies and their families.

Research Support: Provides a rationale for the topic or the use of a particular procedure. Specific research findings are included.

ASSESSMENT BY A DEVELOPMENTAL TEAM

The speech-language pathologist, along with other members of the developmental team, will begin assessment of the child with tracheostomy as soon as the child's health status permits. For children with tracheostomies who are hospitalized in the neonatal intensive care unit, the speech-language pathologist will begin his/her assessment through the use of neurobehavioral assessments. These assessments may be administered by any member of the developmental team who is trained and certified in their use (nurse, occupational therapist, speech-language pathologist, developmental specialist).

Neurobehavioral Assessment

Table 2–2 outlines three neurobehavioral assessments that are commonly used in the assessment of infant behavior (Miller & Quinn Hurst, 1994). The *Neonatal Behavioral Assessment Scale* (*NBAS*; Brazelton, 1984) was developed for the assessment of stable infants of 37 weeks or longer. Norms are available from observations of infants at 3 days of age. There are supplemental items available for use with infants who are at risk. *The Assessment of Preterm Infant Behavior (APIB)* is an extension of the NBAS for the assessment of preterm infants (Als, Lester, Tronick, & Brazelton, 1982). *The Naturalistic Observation of the Preterm Neonate* (*NONB*; Als, 1984) was developed to provide systematic observation of preterm infants who are not capable of sustaining the handling that is required for the administration of the *APIB*.

Each of these assessments requires training on the part of the examiner. The Newborn Individualized Developmental Care and Assessment Program (NIDCAP) has been developed in the United States for the training of health care professionals who work with neonates who are at risk. The program trains professionals to observe neonates, to become proficient at administering the *APIB* and to establish training centers for the *APIB*. Through the training of at least 10% of the nursing staff in NIDCAP procedures, neonatal intensive care units are likely to establish developmental care procedures on a unit-wide basis (Als, 1997). The involvement of at least one parent representative in the NIDCAP training process also aids in the success of establishing developmental care.

The *APIB* and *NONB* are both based on the synactive model of infant behavior described by Als (Als, 1986). The assessments are used to determine how well the infant is functioning in terms of neurobehavioral organization. The level of organization will determine the extent to which the child requires environmental modifications as well as how ready an infant may be for developmental care and intervention. The assessments are used to chart changes in the infant's behavior in response to medical and developmental interventions on a daily basis as well as changes in stability of behavioral organization over time.

TABLE 2–2. Commonly Used Neurobehavioral Infant Assessment Tools

Name of Assessment	*Comments*
The Neonatal Behavioral Assessment Scale (Brazelton, 1984)	Assessment of stable infants of at least 37 weeks gestation Training required
The Assessment of Preterm Infant Behavior (Als, Lester, Tronick, & Brazelton, 1982)	Assessment of preterm infants Handling and positioning of infants required Training required
Naturalistic Observation of the Preterm Neonate (Als, 1984)	Assessment of preterm newborns No handling of infant required Training required

Observation of Signs of Stability and Stress

Observation of infants for signs of stability and stress involves observing various infant subsystems (autonomic, motor, state regulation, and attentional-interactive) (Als, 1986; Table 2–3). Autonomic behaviors involve physiological functioning. Motor behaviors include muscle tone, posture, quality of movement as well as presence of reflexes. State regulation is the regulation of alertness, ranging from deep sleep to fussiness. Attentional-interactive behaviors include the ability to interact with the environment and to take in information. Various behaviors in each area can be observed as indications of the infant's stability (smooth posture, quiet-alert state, regular respiration) or of the infant's stress (arching of the back, changes in color, inability to handle more than one stimulus at a time, difficulty calming after an intervention). By carefully observing the infant, professionals and parents can time interaction to when the child is calm and can withdraw care if the child shows signs of stress. Reduction of interaction when the infant is stressed has helped to reduce the risk of brain hemorrhage and to promote weight gain (Als, Lawhon, Brown, Gibes, Duffy, McAnulty, & Blickman, 1986).

TABLE 2–3. Signs of Stability and Stress in the Infant's Organizational Systems

Systems	*Stability*	*Stress*
Autonomic	Smooth breathing Stable color	Rapid breathing or gasping for breath Pale color
Motor	Good posture Good tone	Hyperflexion of body Arching of back Splaying of fingers
State Regulation	Clear sleep state	Poor sleep Whimpers
Modulation	Robust crying Shows periods of quiet alertness	Glassy eyed, panicky Irritable Slow to transition
Attentional-Interactive	Attends to visual and auditory stimuli	Gaze averted, staring

Note. Adapted from Als, H. (1986). A synactive model of neonatal behavioral organization. Framework of the assessment and support of the neurobehavioral development of the premature infant and his parents in the environment of the neonatal intensive care unit. In J. K. Sweeney (Ed.) The high risk neonate: Developmental therapy perspectives. *Physical and Occupational Therapy in Pediatrics,* 6(3/4), 3–55. Reprinted with permission of Haworth Press, Inc., Binghamton, NY.

ASSESSMENT OF ORAL-MOTOR SKILLS

The speech-language pathologist will also play an important role as a member of the developmental team who assesses a child's oral-motor development and readiness for beginning speech and breast or bottle feeding (Billeaud, 1998). Infants show a gag reflex at 32 weeks gestational age, and the coordination of sucking and swallowing is achieved by most infants who are developing normally at 34 to 35 weeks gestational age. Most infants who are at risk are not breast or bottle fed prior to 34 weeks gestational age. Therefore, many infants who are at risk will be fed by tube for a period of several weeks to several months (or longer in severe cases) prior to oral feedings. Infants are generally required to show stable cardiac and respiratory status and adequate bowel sounds, and to tolerate an oral feed without a major apneic episode prior to initiation of oral feeding on a regular basis (Harris, 1986). Even though the infant will not likely begin oral feeding from the start, many speech-language pathologists and occupational therapists will assess the child's oral-motor skills with the aim of providing early, positive oral experiences.

CONTENT OF GLOBAL ORAL-MOTOR AND FEEDING ASSESSMENT

Box 2–2 outlines the major content areas for oral-motor and feeding assessment of infants. Several researchers and clinicians recommend the use of a global assessment. A global oral-motor assessment combines observation of the infant's oral reflexes and examination for the presence of structural and functional problems with an assessment of the child's organizational responses to oral touch and handling for nonnutritive and nutritive sucking (Glass & Wolf, 1994; Harris, 1986; Sheppard, 1987). Documentation of the child's health history, reason for tracheostomy, and early oral-motor responses within the first month of life will be important in assessing potential structural or sensory factors that may hinder a smooth transition to oral feeding (Arvedson, 1993).

BOX 2–2. Content Areas of Oral-Motor and Feeding Assessment in Infants and Toddlers

- Presence of oral reflexes
- Responses to tactile input
- General level of body motor control and activity
- Physiological control (heart and respiratory rate and respiratory quality in feeding and nonfeeding activities)
- Oral motor control of structures for feeding and speech (lip closure, tongue and jaw movements, strength of suck, rhythmicity of movements)
- Structural integrity of palate, mandible
- Ability to suck on finger, nipple without signs of organizational stress
- Coordination of sucking, swallowing, breathing
- Functionality and adequacy of nonnutritive and nutritive sucking (pleasurable oral experience with ability to take in adequate nutrition in reasonable time period)
- Signs of aspiration or inadequate transfer during swallow

Note. Adapted from Harris, M. (1986). Oral-motor management of the high risk neonate. *Physical and Occupational Therapy in Pediatrics, 6*(3), 231–253. Reprinted with permission of Haworth Press, Inc., Binghamton, NY; and from Wolf, L. S. (1994). A global perspective on feeding assessment in the neonatal intensive care unit. *The American Journal of Occupational Therapy*, *48*(6), 514–526. Reprinted with permission of The American Occupational Therapy Association.

A commonly used descriptive observation tool for oral-motor assessment of infants is the *Neonatal Oral-Motor Assessment Scale (NOMAS)* (Braun & Palmer, 1986). This scale is appropriate for identification of oral-motor behaviors in premature infants at high risk (Case-Smith, Cooper, & Scala, 1989). Table 2–4 identifies several feeding assessments that will be appropriate for assessing oral-motor and feeding behaviors in children.

TABLE 2–4. Instruments for Assessing Oral-motor Functioning and Development of Feeding Skills

Instrument	***Comments***
The Neonatal Oral-Motor Assessment Scale (Braun & Palmer, 1986; revision, Case-Smith, 1988)	Assesses oral-motor and feeding skills in infants
Clinical Feeding Evaluation of Infants (Wolf & Glass, 1992)	Global assessment of reflexes, oral-motor, nutritive sucking, child's responses to touch, nonnutritive and nutritive sucking
Feeding Assessment (Morris & Klein, 1987)	Analyzes development of feeding in relation to the normal developmental sequence, birth to 4 years
Multidisciplinary Feeding Profile (Kenny, Koheil, Greenberg, Reid, Milner, Roman, & Judd, 1989)	Assesses oral reflexes, oral-facial and oral-sensory responses, feeding; appropriate for children with neurological difficulties who do not self-feed

PRESENCE OF FEEDING PROBLEMS

The child with a tracheostomy will not always experience oral-motor and/or feeding difficulties, but may be at risk for such problems. The presence and extent of these difficulties will be influenced by the condition that necessitated the tracheostomy (Arvedson & Brodsky, 1993). If swallowing difficulties are suspected in the child with tracheostomy, a test with myethylene blue should be conducted. Myethylene blue is added to a liquid, and a small amount is given to the child. If the secretions in the tracheal tube are blue, then further examination via modified barium swallow should be considered. See Box 2–3 for the potential impact of tracheostomy and related conditions on oral-motor functioning and feeding.

BOX 2–3. Conditions and Potential Feeding Problems in Children with Tracheostomy

Conditions	Feeding Problems
Tracheostomy/prematurity	Weak suck or incoordination of suck and swallow
Tracheostomy/airway obstruction at or above the level of the larynx	May result in tube feeding; care will be needed to transition a child from tube to oral feeding
Tracheostomy/laryngeal elevation	The weight of the tracheal tube may restrict the elevation of the larynx and influence the adequacy of the pharyngeal swallow (Arvedson, 1993)
Tracheostomy/CNS	Uncoordinated sucking
Tracheostomy/Pierre Robin	Multiple structural difficulties may lead to aspiration, sucking difficulties
Tracheostomy/use of inflated cuff	Inflated cuff against the esophagus may result in swallowing difficulties; oral feeding can take place once deflated cuff is tolerated (Brodsky, 1997)
Tracheostomy/neurological impairment that results in lack of cough or gag or incoordination of suck and swallow	Children who do not exhibit a cough or gag will be fed by tube. Some neurological problems will result in incoordination of suck and swallow

PARENTAL OBSERVATION OF APPROACH AND AVOIDANCE BEHAVIORS

Who? Infant with tracheostomy who is in the intensive care unit.

What? Observation system for describing an infant's responses to stimuli through various approach and avoidance behaviors.

When? The observation system is to be used by parents (working as a team with the speech-language pathologist, or a nurse or social worker) to learn when to approach their child for communication and when to remove stimulation.

Where? In the hospital by parents, caregivers, or selected professionals.

How? Basic instructions that can be easily followed by families are provided.

Why? Observing the child's early responses to stimuli provides the parents with the earliest opportunity to begin to know their infant, to have a specific role in the intensive care unit, and to learn about their infant's basic responses that can be shaped into later communication interactions (VandenBerg, 1993; 1999).

Research Support

Several studies that have evaluated the impact of developmental care on the short-term medical and neurobehavioral outcomes of low-birth-weight children have shown improvements in several medical outcomes for infants. Generally, developmental care has resulted in shorter hospital stays, in shorter time as tube feeders, and in decreases in the number of infants with severe chronic lung disease for experimental versus control group infants (Als, Lawhon, Duffy, McAnulty, Gibes-Grossman, & Blickman, 1994; Fleischer, VandenBerg, Constantinou, Heller, Benitz, Johnson, Rosenthal, & Stevenson, 1995). If the reduction in the severity of lung disease were shown to be a consistent outcome of developmental care in the neonatal intensive care unit, this could have implications for the number of children who may require tracheostomy and/or long-term ventilation.

More recently, researchers have begun to evaluate the effectiveness of specific procedures (physical touch, kangaroo care, etc.) and the effectiveness of parent training programs on medical and developmental outcomes of low-birth-weight children (Als, 1997; Parker, Zahr, Cole, & Brecht, 1992). Although some children with tracheostomy are among the children studied, there are no studies that have focused on the outcome of developmental care in the NICU for children with tracheostomies (Table 2–5).

ASSESSMENT OF DEVELOPMENTAL SKILLS

Once a child's health has stabilized and he/she will tolerate touch and will attend to people, the speech-language pathologist will want to assess the developmental status of the child with tracheostomy. One approach to assessment is to start with a measure that screens for multiple areas of development (play, cognitive, motor, social, and language skills). Several measures that allow for the observation of cognitive and/or play skills in addition to interaction and language skills are: *Assessing Linguistic Behavior* (Olswang, Stoel-Gammon, Coggins, & Carpenter, 1987); *Rossetti Infant-Toddler Language Scale* (Rossetti, 1990); and *The Hawaii Early Learning Profile* (Furuno, O'Reilly, Inatsuka, Husaka, Allmon & Zeisloft-Falbey, 1994). *The Hawaii Early Learning Profile* and the *Rossetti Infant-Toddler Language Scale* have been shown to be widely used by speech-language pathologists for assessing infants in the intensive care unit (Dunn, van Kleeck & Rossetti, 1993b).

The particular developmental assessment instrument that is selected will depend on the setting that is available for assessment, the responsivity of the child, and the amount of time that is available for testing. Some assessments that will provide useful information in multiple areas of development and when time permits more extensive testing are: *The Communication and Symbolic Behavior Scales* (Wetherby & Prizant, 1993); *Assessment, Evaluation, and Programming System* (AEPS; Bricker, 1993); *Transdisciplinary Play Assessment* (Linder, 1993); and *The Carolina Curriculum for Infants and Toddlers-2nd Edition* (Johnson-Martin, Jens, Attermeier, & Hacker, 1991). Several developmental assessments utilize parent reports of the child's behavior and are appropriate for obtaining estimates of ongoing behavior: *Vineland Adaptive Behavior Scales* (Sparrow, Balla, & Cicchetti, 1984); *Ages and Stages Questionnaire (ASQ*; Bricker, Squires, & Mounts, 1995); and *Assessment, Evaluation, and Programming System (AEPS*; Bricker, 1993).

TABLE 2–5. Observing Infant's Approach and Avoidance Behaviors

Approach Behaviors	***My Baby's Cues*** [a]	***What to Do***
Good Color		Stand beside isolette
Regular Respiration		Look into baby's face
Opens Eyes		Let baby hold onto your finger
Fingers or Arms Tucked Towards Body		Softly vocalize
Smooth Movements		(Do one thing at a time and watch for a response)
Good Muscle Tone		
Avoidance Behaviors	***My Baby's Cues*** [a]	***What to Do***
Changes in Color		Move away from the baby
(Pale, Flush)		Stay near, remove eye contact
Changes in Heart Rate or Respiration (Movement of Chest Wall in and out)		Cup hand around baby's feet
Yawning		Place cover over isolette
Hiccuping		
Turns Head Away Flailing of Arms and Legs		(Do one thing at a time and allow the baby time to recover)
Eyes Are Glazed or Baby Staring		
Infant's Ways of Regulating Self	***My Baby's Ways*** [a]	***What to Do***
Sucks on Finger or Pacifier Clasps Hand		Watch for the baby to find his/her own ways to quiet self
Moves Hand to Face		

Note. Adapted from Als, H. (1986). A synactive model of neonatal behavioral organization. Framework of the assessment and support of the neurobehavioral development of the premature infant and his parents in the environment of the neonatal intensive care unit. In J. K. Sweeney (Ed.) The high risk neonate: Developmental therapy perspectives. *Physical and Occupational Therapy in Pediatrics, 6*(3/4), 3–55. Reprinted with permission of Haworth Press, Inc., Binghamton, NY.

[a] = Parents can write their infant's cues or ways in the spaces below

ASSESSING COMPREHENSION AND PLAY SKILLS

Following an assessment of general development, the speech-language pathologist will likely administer other formal or informal measures of receptive language and play skills for several reasons. First, it is important to determine if the child with tracheostomy has receptive language skills that are age appropriate. Second, if the speech-language pathologist recommends a pointing or signing system, it is important to know that the child has the comprehension skills to support the prescribed communication system. The assessment of cognitive skills is important to the speech-language pathologist to determine if the child's receptive and expressive skills are commensurate with the child's cognitive skills. Poor health and early hospitalization may hinder a child's ability to explore objects readily, and some children may fall behind in cognitive as well as receptive language skills. Box 2–4 and Table 2–6 present receptive language and play assessments, respectively, that are appropriate for assessment of children from birth through 3 years.

BOX 2–4. Tests That Assess Language Comprehension, Appropriate for Use with Young Children

Assessment, Evaluation, and Programming System (AEPS; Bricker, 1993)

The Communication and Symbolic Behavior Scales (Wetherby & Prizant, 1993)

The Carolina Curriculum for Infants and Toddlers-2nd Edition (Johnson-Martin, Jens, Attermeier, & Hacker 1991)

MacArthur Communicative Development Inventory (Fenson, Dale, Reznick, Thal, Bates, Hartung, Pethick, & Reilly,1996)

Preschool Language Scale (Zimmerman, Steiner, & Pond, 1992)

Receptive Expressive Emergent Language Scale (Bzoch & League, 1991)

Rossetti Infant Toddler Language Scales (Rossetti,1990)

TABLE 2–6. Assessments for Play Skills, Appropriate for Use with Young Children

Instrument	***Age of Child/Content***
Uzgiris-Hunt Scales of Infant Development (Dunst, 1980)	Birth to 24 months, assesses intentionality, nonverbal cognition
Play Assessment (McCune, 1995)	8 to 30 months, assesses symbolic play skills
Symbolic Play Test-2nd Edition (Lowe & Costello, 1988)	12 to 36 months, assesses symbolic play skills

CHECKLIST OF MAJOR MILESTONES IN RECEPTIVE LANGUAGE FROM BIRTH TO 2 YEARS

Who? Child with tracheostomy whose health has stabilized and who has greater mobility and opportunities to interact.
What? Checklist of Major Milestones in Receptive Language.
When? The observation system is to be used when children are alert and calm.
Where? In the hospital or at home by selected professionals.
How? The observation system can be used by professionals or parents.
Why? Observing the child's receptive language abilities allows the speech-language pathologist to determine the child's level of abilities. Given the limited opportunities to interact with their environment along with the risk of neurological damage, children with tracheostomies are at risk for receptive as well as expressive language delays.

Research Support

Children with tracheostomies generally exhibit stronger receptive than expressive language skills (Simon, Fowler, & Handler, 1983). A closer inspection of the individual language profiles of the 23 children studied following decannulation by Simon et al., 1983 showed that 18/23 subjects exhibited receptive language delays below age expectations (from 2 to 15 months delay) (Table 2–7).

TABLE 2–7. Major Milestones in Receptive Language During the First 2 Years in Children Who Are Developing Normally

Age	*Skill*
1 month	Quiets at sound of familiar voice
3 months	Turns head to sound
4 months	Child recognizes when his/her name is said
5 months	Stops activity when name is called
8 months	Recognizes some common words in familiar context Responds consistently when his/her name is called
10 months	Follows simple directions with increasing accuracy
12 months	Begins to understand simple categories Responds to the word "no" Follows commands accompanied by gestures
15 months	Follows more difficult directions Picks out body parts and articles of clothing from pictures upon request
12–18 months	Understands some words outside familiar routines with contextual cues
18–21 months	Understands "I", "mine" Identifies 15 or more common objects
21–24 months	Understands some two word combinations Will follow a series of commands Develops understanding of action words

Note. Adapted from Rosetti, L. M. (2001). *Communication intervention: Birth to three, second edition*. Albany, NY: Singular Thomson Learning; Stonestreet, R., Jackson, R., & Acton, S. (1991). Guidelines for real partnerships with parents. *Infant Toddler Intevention, 1*, 37.

OBSERVING EARLY COMMUNICATION, SOCIAL, AND COGNITIVE SKILLS

Who? Child with tracheostomy who is exhibiting some responses to the environment and who is functioning developmentally in the 3 to 12 month range.

What? Observation system for describing the early communication, social, and attention skills. A signal is a behavior that a child uses to respond to his/her environment and to show interest and awareness of people and objects.

When? The observation system is to be used when children are alert and calm.

Where? In the hospital or at home by parents, caregivers, or selected professionals.

How? The observation system can be used by parents and professionals. Basic instructions that can be easily followed by families are provided.

Why? Observing the child's early communication and social cues helps parents and professionals to understand the child's early ways of communicating, to note the child's readiness for treatment, and to increase expectations for communication by realistic increments. The goal of observation is to determine the primary early signals used by children with tracheostomy.

Research Support

Because some children with tracheostomy may not vocalize at all or may not initiate communication frequently, it is important that parents notice and respond to the child's communication and social attempts when they occur (Adamson & Dunbar, 1991). It has been shown that responsiveness on the part of parents and caregivers increases intentional communication (Yoder, Warren, McCathren, & Leew, 1998).

Background

The communication, social, and cognitive skills exhibited by the child reflect the child's awareness of his/her surroundings. Parents, health care staff, and developmental specialists, who have the earliest contact and opportunities to communicate with the child, will want to pay attention to communication attempts by children with tracheostomies. Any attempts to interact with others should be encouraged and may be reinforced and shaped into more sophisticated communicative signals and turn-taking exchanges (Table 2–8).

TABLE 2–8. Outline of Early Communication, Social, and Cognitive Skills

Age	*Conversational Skills*	*Social Skills*	*Cognitive Skills*
3 months	Smiles at person talking; protests by vocalizing; uses consistent signals for hunger, distress, pleasure	Stops crying when touches bottle; can be comforted by talking, holding, rocking	Anticipates reoccurring daily caretaking activities
6 months	Requests ongoing action of familiar activity through body movement, eye contact; coordinated looking and listening	Smiles reciprocally, attracts attention by making sounds, eye contact	Anticipates frequently occurring events in nursery rhymes after several exposures
9 months	Uses gaze to select conversational partner; changes pitch and volume to signify intensity	Participates in simple games Repeats activity that gets reaction from adults	Anticipates frequently occurring events in games on first trial
12 months	Raises arms to be picked up; engages in reciprocal turn-taking	Gives items upon request Imitates game playing	Remembers location of objects placed there a few seconds ago
15 months	Uses gestures—"all gone," "so big," uses words, signs to express wants	Shares with adults; shows affection	Reacts to change in familiar game or routine

Note. Adapted from Johnson-Martin, N. M., Jens, G., Attermeier, M. & Hacker, J. (1991). *The Carolina Curriculum for Infants and Toddlers with Special Needs*, (49–57) Paul H. Brookes Publishing Co. Reprinted with permission from Paul H. Brookes Publishing Co., Baltimore.

Procedures and Instructions:

Watch and Become Familiar with Each Child

Begin by watching for any of the behaviors listed on the checklist or similar behaviors shown by the child. Watch for times of day or activities where the child seems alert. Try to interact with him or her at those times. Note the situation or time of day when the child exhibits awareness of persons or objects.

Watch and Respond When the Child Does Something

Next, notice if some behaviors occur more frequently than others. Observe the child for a set period of time and note the number of times that the child exhibits a particular behavior. Or try to elicit eye, hand, or mouth movements. When the child communicates, imitate or comment on what he/she does. Keep track of what you do and what the child does in response. Responding helps your child to know that you acknowledge what he/she has done.

Watch for More Sophisticated Signals

As the child becomes more consistent in using some behaviors, notice if the communication signals progress to more sophisticated levels. For example, a child's smiling at a person when talking (3-month skill) advances to coordinated looking and listening at 6 months of age.

OBSERVING A CHILD'S ABILITY TO VOCALIZE

Who? A child with tracheostomy who has not been observed to produce sound.
What? Procedure for determining if a child is capable of producing sound while tracheostomized.
When? The procedure should be employed when the child produces poor, weak vocalizations or when the child is not known to vocalize. Some children may produce spontaneous vocalizations if air leaks around the tracheal tube. Many children with tracheostomies may be 7–8 months of age before they vocalize on a consistent basis (Driver, 2000). Various factors may contribute to the child's ability to vocalize, including the stability of the child's health, sufficient growth to allow for air leakage around the cannula, adequate health and airway status to support use of a speaking valve.
Where? In a place where the child feels comfortable in the hospital or at home by the speech-language pathologist.
How? Instructions for how to use the procedure are provided.
Why? It is important to know if facilitating vocalizations is a realistic treatment goal or if an alternative nonverbal system needs to be instituted as a current means of communication.

Research Support

A child's ability to vocalize and be able to feel and hear his/her own vocalizations is thought to be essential for future speech production (Bleile, 1998; Locke & Pearson, 1992). Children with tracheostomies need opportunities to practice speech production skills once they can create airflow around the tracheal tube or through a speaking valve.

Procedures:

Gathering Information

1. Ask the parent or caregiver if the child has been observed to vocalize. Ask if any audible vocalizations have occurred when the child cries (vocalizing sometimes will accompany the effortful act of crying).
2. Check the child's medical records for the length of time since the tracheotomy. Children who have recently undergone tracheostomy may have a tracheal tube that is tightly fitted and does not allow for any leakage of air around the tube. Swelling of tracheal tissue may make it uncomfortable for the child to occlude the stoma and create pressure to allow air to escape around the tracheal tube. Confirm with the otolaryngologist that the child has the capacity to produce air and vocalize. Review the medical record for specific information relative to the severity of airway compromise. This information can help the speech-language pathologist to determine the child's potential to vocalize.
3. For the child who has been observed to make sounds under some conditions attempt to elicit vocalizations from the child. Ask the parents to demonstrate for you how they have elicited any vocalizations from their child.

Specific Procedures for Eliciting Vocalizing:

1. Place the child in an upright position to facilitate adequate breath support for vocalization. Some children will have more success on their tummies (this position wll bring the chin and tongue forward and/or provide more support for some children, depending on their head support and motor strength).
2. Create a positive and motivating situation for speaking.
   - Use reactive toys such as a Busy Bee toy or Jack-in-the-box with pop-up animals that might motivate the child to squeal or vocalize.
   - Use See and Say toys where the child might try to imitate the sound of one of the animals.
   - Use toys that are likely to get the child to open his/her mouth to vocalize or show excitement.
3. Once you have interested the child in a speaking situation or toy, attempt to slowly and carefully occlude the child's stoma with a gloved finger and allow the child an opportunity to vocalize on expiration. Make sure that occlusion occurs following inspiration and is prior to expiration. Place toys at or above eye level so the child will need to reach or look up. This will allow the speech-language pathologist to more readily occlude the stoma (if the child is looking down, the stoma is not easily accessible).
4. Occlude the stoma for a second or two and see if the child will blow air or make a sound. Watch the child for signs of respiratory distress (changes in skin color, signs of discomfort or fright, signs of labored breathing, increased respiratory rate). Frequently, the speech-language

pathologist works with the respiratory therapist when getting children to vocalize the first few times. The respiratory therapist can monitor the child for signs of distress as well as make sure that all equipment is properly connected. It is important that the child associates positive experiences with vocalizing, so if the child becomes distressed, stop the activity and try it again at another time.

5. If the child shows no indications of vocalizing, check to ensure that the child is anatomically capable of vocalizing. If there are no complications to hinder vocalizing, keep trying on a regular basis to get the child to vocalize.

6. The child who is able to vocalize while occluding his/her stoma is considered a good candidate for a speaking valve and/or for engaging in vocal turn-taking with an occluded stoma (Silverman McGowan, Bleile, Fus, & Barnas, 1993).

ASSESSING NONVERBAL AND VERBAL MEANS OF COMMUNICATION

Children with tracheostomies may remain in the prelinguistic stage of communication (i.e., communicating through nonverbal means and with sounds) and rely on nonverbal means of communicating (i.e., facial expressions, head movements, gaze, and/or gestures) for an extended period of time. They may use gestures and facial expressions at an age when children who have had a full range of opportunities and means to communicate are using words and word combinations. Children with tracheostomies may also use more unconventional means of communicating (their communication is nonspecific or difficult to interpret) than children who have had opportunities to communicate through verbal as well as nonverbal means.

Box 2–5 outlines major ways children under 3 years of age who are tracheostomized during the prelinguistic stage are likely to communicate. The communication means range from facial expressions and head and body movements to more elaborate gestures and manual signs. Verbal means of communicating range from the ability to make sounds to the production of more sophisticated, recognizable consonants and words. The communication means may be conventional or unconventional as well as intentional or unintentional (Bates, Camaioni, & Volterra, 1975; Owens, 1996).

BOX 2–5. Means of Communication

- Use of facial expressions, head and body movements
- Creation of voicing or sound
- Use of specific vowels or consonants
- Use of gestures
- Use of words
- Use of manual signs
- Use of augmentative system to express needs, concepts (pointing to pictures, activating a touch talk system)

OBSERVING NONVERBAL IMITATION

The child with tracheostomy may exhibit splintered imitation skills. Many children with tracheostomies will be slow to imitate vocalizations, but some will imitate sounds (tongue clicks, lip smacks, raspberries). All children with tracheostomies, who do not have motor difficulties, will imitate nonverbal limb movements. Table 2–9 reviews selected nonverbal activities and the age of acquisition for these activities from "A Method for Describing Interaction Styles of Handicapped Prelanguage Children" (Norris & Hoffman, 1990).

TABLE 2–9. Development of Nonverbal Imitation in Prelanguage Children Who have Handicaps, 7–24 months.

Limb Actions	*Vocalizations*	*Facial and Body Postures*
Level III. 7–9 months		
Imitates movements (waving arm, patting hand on tray)	Attempts to imitate speech sounds & CV sequences (may not be same as adult model)	Smiles or laughs when teased or entertained Pulls back or moves to reject something
Pushes away unwanted items	Vocalizations show pitch, quality, intensity, etc. changes	Uses eye contact to indicate recurrence or help
Moves limbs to indicate reactivation or recurrence		Moves by leaning over or forward to follow the actions of adults or objects
Grabs adult's fingers or pulls adult's hand to indicate recurrence	Vocalizes to have toy reactivated or adult do action	
Does action for familiar games (pat-a-cake)	Vocalizes at object, looks to adult, indicates need for help by pulling	
	Imitates nonspeech sounds (coughs, smacking lips)	
	Imitates words without attaching meaning	
	Babbles phrases with 4 or more different syllables	
Level IV. 10–12 months		
Points to noticed objects	Repeats vocalization if responded to	Wiggles body to continue action (bouncing)
Points to parts of objects upon imitation	Fusses, cries when desired object removed	Moves body to represent action (rocking for rocking toy)
Imitates actions that are functional or repeats modeled action to make event recur	Expresses negative reaction through vocalization Uses single word to label	
Imitates novel gesture	Imitates a series of sounds said by the adult	
Extends toy to give, but doesn't release	Uses jargon to toys, people as if talking	
Gestures to represent an action		
Uses social gestures like bye-bye		

(continues)

TABLE 2–9. *(continued)*

Limb Actions	*Vocalizations*	*Facial and Body Postures*
Level V. 13–18 months		
Gives object to adult to (re)activate toy	Uses five words Uses one word for many meanings	Imitates facial movement or expression Leads adults by hand to desired object
Points, reaches, etc. to object to indicate wanting them	Imitates variety of words Uses jargon mixed with real words	
Repeats actions that produce laughter or attention		
Uses gestures in combination to indicate wants		
Level VI. 19–24 months		
Hands objects to adult to be shared (or book to be read)	Vocabulary of 10–50 words Imitates 2–3 word combinations	Does own actions if other person will not respond
Does a series of relational actions	Trys to describe experiences using jargon mixed with real words	
	Uses variety of word classes (action, agent, attributes, etc.)	

Note. Adapted from Norris, J. A. & Hoffman, P. R. (1990). Comparison of adult-initiated vs. child initiated interaction styles with handicapped prelanguage children. *Language, Speech and Hearing Services in Schools*, 21, pp. 28–36. Reprinted with permission of the American Speech-Language-Hearing Association and the author.

OBSERVING COMMUNICATION MEANS AND INTENTIONS

Who? The child with tracheostomy who is exhibiting some responses to the environment and is functioning developmentally in the 0 to 13 month range.

What? Observation system for describing stages in a child's use of nonverbal and verbal communication means and the intentions adults are likely to attribute to those communication attempts.

When? The observation system is to be used when children are alert and calm. The observations should be employed for a set length of time (10 minutes) during several activities and take place on three or more occasions.

Where? In the hospital or at home by professionals and/or parents.

How? Professionals should observe interactions between the child and a familiar adult.

Why? Children generally use a variety of communication means to communicate and gradually move from unintentional means to intentional means of communicating at 8 to 9 months of age. The means of communication used to express a variety of intentions are also important. Children communicate for purposes of regulating others' behavior, to be social, and to maintain joint attention. These communication intentions are important to later language development. Children with tracheostomies may be restricted in both communication means and intentions. Some children may express a variety of intentions through a smaller number of means.

Research Support

Young children from 8 to 13 months communicate for three basic reasons: to regulate their own and other's behavior, to socialize with others, and to establish joint attention. Communicating for these basic reasons has been shown to be important to the development of future language skills (Wetherby, Cain, Yonclas, & Walker, 1988; Wetherby & Prutting, 1984; Wetherby & Prizant, 1993). Some children with tracheostomies have shown good skills in communicating to regulate the behavior of others, but communicated less frequently for social reasons or to establish joint attention (Kertoy, & Waters, 1995).

Background

Table 2–10 provides information about both communication means and potential interpretations of the intentions of the child's communication during the earliest developmental stages (from 3 to 13 months) (Weitzman, 1992). The table also outlines the infants transition from unintentional to intentional communication. Unconventional signals are attempts to affect another's behavior, but the specific or intended meaning may not be clear to the receiver (i.e., whining, squirming). Conventional gestures or vocalizations are used to communicate a meaning that is easier for the receiver to interpret (pointing to a specific object). Communication means may be intentional or unintentional. Intentional communication is marked by one or more identifiable characteristics. The child directs his/her gaze at an object and then at a person. If the attempt is misinterpreted, the child is likely to repeat or modify the communication attempt. In children with normally developing language, intentional means of communication begin at 8 or 9 months of age, and the child's communication becomes more conventional as well. Unintentional communication attempts may be given meaning by the adult (e.g., the child whines and the adult says, "Oh, you must be hungry.").

TABLE 2–10. First Three Stages of Communication and Language Development

Stage/Age/Description	*How the Infant Behaves*	*Caregiver's Interpretation of Why the Infant is Communicating*
Stage 1		
Birth to 3 months	Cries, fusses, looks or moves away	To protest, reject, show distress/displeasure
The infant communicates reflexively	Looks, smiles, makes vowel-like sounds	To request action/object
	Looks, makes sounds, smiles, makes body movements, voice changes (loudness and pitch)	To respond to/show awareness of, and interest in, others
Stage 2		
3 to 8 months	Cries, fusses, looks or moves away	To protest, reject, show distress/displeasure
The infant is interested in others, but doesn't communicate intentionally	Looks at what/whom he/she wants, reaches, moves towards others, makes a variety of consonant and vowel sounds	To request action/object
	Looks at person, makes sounds, smiles, body movements, changes loudness and pitch	To respond to/show awareness of, and interest in, others
	Makes sounds or performs action related to routine, e.g., rocks back and forth to request "Row, Row, Row Your Boat"	To request social play routine (New)
	Looks, makes sounds, babbles, e.g., "gagaga," changes loudness and pitch, smiles, makes body movements	To call for attention (New)

(continues)

TABLE 2–10. *(continued)*

Stage/Age/Description	***How the Infant Behaves***	***Caregiver's Interpretation of Why the Infant is Communicating***
Stage 3		
8 to 13 months	Cries, moans	To direct or control another's behavior
The infant communicates intentionally and becomes very social	Requests action/object	Protests Points, gestures To interact for social purposes
	Requests social routine	Pantomimes
	Calls for attention	Uses sounds that have special meaning
	Requests comfort	
	Shows off	Makes eye contact
	Greets	
	Uses combinations of pointing, looking and making sounds	To establish joint attention (new) Draws attention to objects/events/people in environment
	Single words	Labels
		Requests information

Note. Taken from Weitzman, E. (1992). *Learning Language and Loving It* (Toronto: Hanen Center, pp. 49–55). Reprinted with permission from The Hanen Centre, Toronto, Ontario.

Procedures:

This form can be modified to fit the ways the child you are observing communicates. Write in the common ways that the child communicates. Observe if the child communicates for a variety of reasons. Also note if the child has ample opportunities to communicate. The communication partners will play an important role in creating an environment in which the child is expected to communicate (see the next section).

OBSERVING THE COMMUNICATION ENVIRONMENT

The speech-language pathologist will want to carefully examine the extent to which the child's environment affords opportunities for learning receptive and expressive language skills. Because parents and caregivers begin early interactions with medically fragile infants cautiously and limit the intensity of stimuli, this pattern may be carried into the period when the child is capable of additional stimulation. The language skills of children with tracheostomies may be underestimated at home and in the hospital. Parents and professionals alike may assume that a child cannot perform a particular task. Indeed, the child may be capable of performing more skills, but is not given opportunities to exhibit or practice those skills. Professionals should ask the following types of questions about the child's environment.

Guidelines

1. Is the environment encouraging or hindering language development?
2. Is the child offered choices on a regular basis and expected to express his or her needs?
3. Do parents and caregivers routinely label objects and actions for the child? Do they engage in parallel talk and make comments on activities as they occur?
4. Is there a typical time as well as set routines for feeding, dressing, and bathing? Does the child have routines so that he or she can recognize the steps in reoccurring, daily events and learn to anticipate upcoming events?
5. Is the child regularly given opportunities to play with appropriate toys that will improve motor or cognitive skills, to achieve the next higher level? Are labels provided for the objects or instructions/demonstrations provided for what to do with particular objects?

OBSERVING EARLY GESTURES

Who? Child with tracheostomy whose health has stabilized, who is gaining weight, and who has greater mobility and opportunities to communicate.
What? Observation system for monitoring gesture use.
When? The observation system is to be used when children are alert and calm.
Where? In the hospital or at home by parents, caregivers, or selected professionals.
How? The observation system can be used by parents and professionals. Instructions for how to use the system are provided.
Why? Observing the child's early gestures helps parents and professionals to understand how the child is conceptualizing the world and if the child appears to have the nonlinguistic skills that frequently coincide with the onset of speech (Bates, Thal, Whitesell, Fenson, & Oakes, 1989).

Research Support

The use of single, recognitory gestures has been linked to the onset of word use in children who are developing language normally (Thal, Tobias, & Morrison, 1991). A recognitory gesture is a gesture in which the function of an object is depicted through an action completed with the object or an empty word (e.g., pretending to eat with a fork) (Thal & Bates, 1988). Some children who are late to talk show an overreliance on gestures. Late talkers may be similar in gesture use to children with tracheostomies because both groups of children are communicating by means other than through word use for a longer period of development than children who are developing language normally (Thal & Tobias, 1994). The use of multiple gestures in context has been linked to the ability to combine words (Thal, Tobias, & Morrison, 1991). Gesture use is important to the practicing speech-language pathologists because it is an indication that children, including children with tracheostomies, have the skills to refer to objects, an important skill in the development of early language (Bates, et al. 1989).

Background

Several checklists and assessments are available for observing the number and kinds of gestures used by young children, including those with tracheostomies. Several procedures will be proposed and explained. A gesture checklist based on the development of gestures outlined by Iverson and Thal (1998) will be presented because approximate ages for the use of gestures in children who are developing language normally have been specified by these authors and provide useful guidelines for the speech-language pathologist who is working with the child with tracheostomy. In addition, a procedure for eliciting recognitory gestures is provided as this procedure would be relatively easy for the speech-language pathologist to administer. In addition, the use of recognitory gestures is important to the onset of word use in children (Bates, et al., 1989; Thal & Tobias, 1994). Finally, an explanation of the gesture categories from the *Communicative Development Inventories: Words and Gestures* (*CDI*; Fenson, Dale, Reznick, Thal, Bates, Hartung, Pethick, & Reilly, 1996) is provided. The advantage of using the *CDI: Words and Gestures* as a measure of gesture use is that norms are available on the use of gestures in children with normally developing language (Fenson et al., 1996), in children who are late to talk (Thal & Tobias, 1994), and in children with tracheostomies (Kertoy & Morrison, 2000) (Table 2–11).

TABLE 2–11. Development of Gesture Types in Normally Developing Children and Approximate Age of Onset

Behavior	*Age Range of Onset*	*Check If Observed*
Use eye gaze to draw attention to object	12 months	
Joint attention to object with adult	12 months	
Use of deictic gestures (establish reference)		
Giving	8–14 months	
Showing	8–14 months	
Reaching	8–14 months	
Pointing	12–14 months	
	(These gestures continue to increase with word use)	
Use of representational gestures (establish reference and carry specific semantic content)	11–16 months (These gestures decline between 16–20 months with word use)	
Object related—flapping arms to show airplane		
Culturally defined conventional—waving bye		
Overlap of gesture and word use	14 months and later	

Note. Adapted from Iverson, J. and Thal, D. (1998). Communicative transitions: There's more to the hand than meets the eye, In S. F. Warren and J. Reichle (Eds.) *Transitions in prelinguistic communication*. pp. 59–86. Baltimore: Paul H. Brookes Publishing. Reprinted with permission of Brookes Publishing Co.

USE OF SPONTANEOUS AND IMITATED RECOGNITORY GESTURES

Who? The child of approximately 8 months and older with tracheostomy with adequate head and trunk support to reach for and handle objects.

What? A procedure for eliciting the spontaneous use of recognitory gestures. Recognitory gestures are action schemes carried out with familiar toys or household objects (e.g., brushing hair with a brush) (Bates, et al., 1989). These gestures serve to establish reference and are called recognitory. Children will use these action schemes with the actual object and then later complete the action without the object or with a substitute object.

When? Used when the speech-language pathologist would like to know the extent of a child's ability to gesture with objects.

Where? Procedure can be used at home or in the hospital by the speech-language pathologist.

How? The procedure includes instructions.

Why? The child with tracheostomy may not have had adequate exposure to a variety of toys and objects nor opportunity to manipulate them. Findings from the procedure will help the speech-language pathologist in planning activities to stimulate receptive language and cognitive experiences related to understanding and manipulating objects.

Research Support

Thal and Tobias (1994) studied imitative and spontaneous use of recognitory gestures in three groups of children: late talkers, language-matched controls, and age/comprehension-matched controls. Thal and Tobias (1994) found that late talkers (18.6 to 33 months) and language matched controls (11.2 to 20.8 months) spontaneously used more recognitory gestures than verbal labels, as compared to the age/comprehension-matched controls (18.3 to 33.2 months), who used a similar number of recognitory gestures and verbal labels. Late talkers and age/comprehension-matched controls imitated similar numbers of recognitory gestures. Both late talkers and age-matched controls found it easier to produce recognitory gestures with real objects and supportive language than with placeholder objects (a block that stood for another object) and neutral language than the language-matched controls (Table 2–12).

TABLE 2–12. Procedure for Eliciting Spontaneous Use of Recognitory Gestures

Objects	*Associated Gesture*
toy cup	drink
toy airplane	fly
toy car	roll
toy doll	hug
toy dog	walk
toy flower	sniff
real toothbrush	brush teeth
real spoon	eat
toy phone	receiver to ear
real hat	put hat on head

Note. From Bates, E., Thal, D., Whitesell, K., Fenson, L & Oakes, L. (1989). Integrating language and gesture in infancy. pp. 1019. *Developmental Psychology, 25*(6), 1004–1019. Reprinted with permission of the author and the American Psychological Association, Inc.

Instructions:

Present child with the above 10 objects, one at a time. Allow the child to play with the object for 30 seconds. If the child does not produce a recognitory gesture, the speech-language pathologist should ask, "What do you do with that?" (Bates, Thal, Whitesell, Fenson, & Oakes 1989; Thal & Tobias, 1994).

TYPES OF GESTURES MEASURED BY *THE COMMUNICATIVE DEVELOPMENT INVENTORIES: WORDS AND GESTURES*

Who? The child with tracheostomy from 8 to 16 months of age or older children with gesture use in the age range of 8 to16 months.

What? Types of gestures measured by *The Communicative Development Inventories: Words and Gestures*.

When? When the speech-language pathologist is interested in knowing the number and types of gestures used by a child.

Where? At home or in a quiet room in the hospital or clinic.

How? The parent completes the checklist. The checklist can be completed over a period of time. The parent indicates with a check the gestures that the child has been observed to use. The manual for the *CDI: Words and Gestures* includes complete instructions on how the checklist is to be completed. The speech-language pathologist may use only the gesture section from the *CDI: Words and Gestures*, as norms are provided for each section of the inventories. The *CDI: Words and Gestures* may be used with children who are older than the upper-age limits of the inventories when the speech-language pathologist wants to assess a child's strengths and weaknesses. The authors of the inventories advise the speech-language pathologist not to use the *CDI: Words and Gestures* if a child's score is above the median score for 16 months on the inventories because this practice may result in an underestimation of the child's language abilities (Fenson, Dale, Reznick, Thal, Bates, Hartung, Pethick, & Reilly, 1996, pg. 25).

Why? The *CDI: Words and Gestures* has been normed for use with children 0–16 months of age. The norms make it easy for the speech-language pathologist to determine if a child's gestures are age appropriate and if a child is using a variety of gesture types.

Research Support

Kertoy and Morrison (2000) studied gesture use in two children with tracheostomies in place who had opportunities to vocalize. Subject 1, at 26 months and a comprehension level of 137 words on the *CDI*, used 13 early (Categories A and B) and 22 late gestures (Categories C, D, and E; refer to Table 2–13 for types of gestures). Subject 2, at 19 months and a comprehension level of 137 words, used 12 early gestures (Categories A and B) and 19 late gestures (Categories C, D, and E) on the *CDI*. Both of these children used fewer late gestures in Categories D and E than late talkers with similar word comprehension skills at a mean age of 15.9 months (Thal & Tobias, 1994).

TABLE 2–13. Gesture Types Assessed with the *Communicative Development Inventories: Words and Gestures* (Fenson, et al., 1996)

Category	*Category Type*	*No. of Items*	*Example*
Early/A	First Communicative	12	Nods head "yes"
Early/B	Games and Routines	6	Plays patty cake
Late/C	Actions with Objects	17	Combs or brushes own hair
Late/D	Pretending to Be a Parent	13	Feeds with bottle (stuffed animal)
Late/E	Imitating Other Adult Actions	15	Puts key in lock or door

Note. Categories based on *Communicative Development Inventories: Words and Gestures* (L. Fenson, P. S. Dale, J. S. Reznick, D. Thal, E. Bates, J. P. Hartung, S. Pethick & J. S. Reilly,1996). San Diego: Singular Publishing Group.

WAYS OF ASSESSING VOCALIZATIONS

The assessment of a child's ability to vocalize is an important aspect of a communication assessment for the child with tracheostomy. The ability to vocalize and hear one's own vocalizations is thought to be important in fostering speech production in young children. The ability of the child to vocalize at all, will have implications for the type of communication system that the speech-language pathologist and family ultimately select for the child.

An assessment of a child's ability to vocalize and observations of the vocalizations may include several measures: (a) a child's awareness of producing sounds and ability to produce any sound, (b) the types of vocalizations produced as appropriate to a child's age, (c) the amount of talking, and (d) the complexity of syllable structures. These assessments will likely be completed on a serial basis to note anatomical or developmental changes that will be reflected in changes in rate, type, or complexity of vocalizations.

ANALYZING THE RATE OF VOCALIZING

Who? The child with tracheostomy who is beginning to vocalize and for whom the speech-language pathologist would like to increase the amount of vocalizing.
What? Procedure for counting the number of spontaneous vocalizations per minute.
When? When the child is beginning to vocalize. Record the number of vocalizations the child produces at the same time each day or during the same activity for a specific length of time (10 minutes) for each sample.
Where? At home or in the hospital or clinic in a location where the child is comfortable.
How? The speech-language pathologist should record the child with a portable tape recorder and microphone of good quality or lend a recorder to the child's family.
Why? The amount of talking has been associated with positive gains in later language development (Locke, 1998). Those children who talk and engage in interaction with others appear to have more opportunities to learn language than those children who are reticent and rarely interact with others.

Research Support

Locke and Pearson (1990) showed that one child who was tracheostomized from age 1;5 to 1;8 (years; months) vocalized 1.81 spontaneous utterances per minute. This rate increased to 6.4 utterances per minute from age 1;8 to 1;9 (years; months) once the child was decannulated.

Procedures:

1. Record and count the number of separate and spontaneous vocalizations that occur in a set period of time (10 minutes). (For the child who vocalizes infrequently, the period of time may need to be increased to 20 minutes to obtain an appropriate sample). Spontaneous utterances are those utterances that do not occur in direct response to an adult's cue or question. Camp, Morgan, and Schmidt (1987) calculated the rate of vocalizing by noting the number of nondistress, nonrespiratory vocalizations separated by at least a momentary pause (taking a breath). They calculated the number of "vocalizing units" occurring during a 5-minute observation period in children 4 to 6 months of age.
2. Obtain several speech samples of equal lengths of time for each child's vocalizations. An appropriate sampling procedure might include samples taken prior to treatment, several samples taken during treatment, and several samples obtained following treatment. Also samples could be obtained while a child was tracheostomized and then for a period of time after decannulation to note gradual increases in vocalization once the child is decannulated. Finally, samples could be taken prior to the placement of a speaking valve and then over regular intervals while the speaking valve is worn.
3. Divide the number of spontaneous utterances that occurred in a sample by the number of minutes in the sample. Obtain the number of vocalizations per minute.

PERCENTAGE AND TYPES OF VOCALIZATIONS

Who? The child with tracheostomy who has been vocalizing on his/her own with the stoma occluded or with the aid of a speaking valve or electrolarynx (a small electrolarynx held by the speech-language pathologist may allow the child to feel the vibrations and help him/her to start vocalizing).

What? Types of vocalizations and the percentage of each type.

When? The procedure could be used when the speech-language pathologist wants to learn if the child's utterances are showing a normal developmental progression that many children follow during the babbling and early words periods.

Where? Observe the child when the child is likely to vocalize and in several different situations or activities to ensure that a representative sample of a child's abilities has been obtained.

How? Collect multiple samples of equal lengths of time.

Why? Children who are developing normally go through a natural progression of using mainly vowels (2–4 months) to producing a limited number of consonants to the using 11–12 different consonants by age 4–6 months (Proctor, 1989; Stoel-Gammon & Otomo, 1986).

Research Support

Locke and Pearson (1990) showed that one child with tracheostomy exhibited an average of 4.3 different consonant segments (range 3–6 different consonants) at age 1:8 to 1:9 (years:months). Stoel Gammon and Otomo (1986) showed that the number of different consonants increased with age in 11 hearing babies, from 11.3 different consonants at age 4 to 6 months to an average of 29.5 different consonants at age 16 to 18 months.

Kertoy and Morrison (2000) showed that two subjects, with tracheostomies in place and with opportunities to vocalize, used fewer different consonants than the numbers reported by Stoel-Gammon and Otomo (1986). Subject 1, at 21 months, had a phonetic inventory containing 5 different consonants while Subject 2, at 17 months, had a phonetic inventory containing 7 different consonants.

Instructions:

Note the number of vocalizations used by the child. Categorize each vocalization into one of the categories (vowel only, vowel + velar or glottal, vowel + nasal or stop, vowel + other consonant). Calculate the percentage of utterances out of the total utterances that contain a vowel only. The speech-language pathologist should expect to see a higher percentage of utterances that contain only vowels in the beginning. The percentage of utterances with only vowels should decrease over time and be replaced by utterances with one or more consonants (Morrison, 1998). Children with tracheostomies have been shown to follow a normal developmental sequence, but the attainment of milestones is much slower than in children who are developing language normally (Kertoy & Morrison, 2000; Morrison, 1998).

SEQUENCE OF SOUND DEVELOPMENT

Several detailed sequences of sound production have been published, and the reader is encouraged to locate these in the resource section and to use these sequences as appropriate. For many children with tracheostomies, the major milestones in the developmental sequence will initially be the predominant use of vowels and a few consonants and, gradually, the use of different consonants. Vowels are produced with an open vocal tract, while consonant production requires some degree of constriction of the vocal tract. In order to produce consonants, the child needs to control the stream of air within the mouth as well as to coordinate the articulators to create the type of constriction (manner of articulation) in a particular location (place of articulation) (Kent, 1998). The reader is provided with a simple sequence of sound development including those developments that will likely be most crucial for the child with tracheostomy (See Form 2–1). The ages at which children who are developing language typically reach these milestones are also included (Bleile & Miller, 1994, Paul, 1995).

FORM 2–1. Types of Vocalizations and Age of Onset

Check Child's Primary Type	***Vocalization Type(s)***	***Age of Onset***
_______	Use of vowels	Birth to 2 months
_______	Use of vowels primarily, and use of glottal or velar consonants	2 to 4 months
_______	Use of consonants increases including use of front stops or nasals	4 to 6 months
_______	Use of number of different consonants increases	6 to 10 months
_______	Use of raspberries, lip smacks	
_______	Use of variations in pitch	
_______	Production of CV syllable	
_______	Reduplication of CV or CVCV	
_______	Utterances produced with full stop consonants	
_______	CV or CVC produced with a variety of consonants	10 to 12 months
_______	Variegated babbling (syllables are not identical)	
_______	Approximations of single words occur	

Note. Adapted from Proctor, A. (1989). Stages of noncry vocal development in infancy: A protocol for assessment. *Topics in Language Disorders, 10*(1), 26–42. Reprinted with permission of Aspen Publishers, Inc. Gaithersburg, MD.

PHONETIC INVENTORY OF CONSONANT USE

Who? Child with tracheostomy in place who has had some experience vocalizing or the child who has been recently decannulated and is vocalizing. The child is producing vowels and beginning to use consonants.
What? A procedure for completing a phonetic inventory.
When? Completion of an inventory is appropriate when a child is beginning to use consonants and is capable of producing at least 20 speech-like vocalizations (Stoel-Gammon and Otomo, 1986).
Where? In the hospital or in the home by the speech-language pathologist.
How? Completion of a phonetic inventory is done by the speech-language pathologist. Instructions for how to complete an inventory are provided.
Why? The size and content of the phonetic inventory has been shown to be a good predictor of later language development (Stoel-Gammon, 1992).

Research Support

Stoel-Gammon (1985) has shown that the number of phones in a child's phonetic inventory increases from 15 to 24 months in normally developing children and that the the size of the inventory is associated with later language developments (Stoel-Gammon, 1992). The phonetic inventories of several children following decannulation have been shown be smaller than would be expected in normally developing children at similar ages, but there is a rapid increase in the number of consonants used in the months following decannulation (Bleile, 1998).

Procedures:

1. Phonetic inventories are generally completed when children are capable of producing 10 different words in a 1-hour period and when the child is in the 10 to 50 word period of language development.
2. Count spontaneous, not imitated productions.
3. Include the sounds contained in each word only once. If the same word occurs a second time and is pronounced differently, the second production may also be included in the analysis.
4. Single phones that occur in a given position in at least two different words are included in a child's inventory.
5. Allophones are considered exemplars of the target phone.
6. Count the phones that occur in both initial and final positions.
7. Some children with tracheostomies may not produce enough utterances or words initially to meet the criteria established by Stoel-Gammon (1985) for use with normally developing children from 15 to 24 months of age.
8. Stoel-Gammon and Otomo (1986) used less stringent criteria when completing phonetic inventories for children with normal hearing of 4 to 18 months, and for children with hearing loss 4 to 28 months.
9. The child should produce at least 20 speech-like vocalizations.
10. Obtain multiple speech samples from each child.
11. Count the number of different consonants in each sample.

12. Include each different consonant and the number of times it occurs.

13. Consonants other than w, j, and h are considered true consonants, and only true consonants were included by Stoel-Gammon and Otomo (1986).

CALCULATING THE PERCENTAGE OF CANONICAL SYLLABLES

Who? The child who has been recently decannulated and who can vocalize or a child with tracheostomy who can vocalize (around the tracheal tube, by covering the stoma or by using a speaking valve).
What? A procedure for calculating the percentage of canonical syllables produced in a speech sample.
When? The speech-language pathologist would use this procedure to document changes in consonant and syllable use. It is appropriate for the child who is capable of vocalizing regularly and producing consonants. It will show the child who is comfortable with producing CV or VC or more complex syllables. It emphasizes the use of consonants within the syllable as opposed to the complexity of the structure (see next procedure).
Where? May be employed at home or in the hospital where the child is comfortable vocalizing.
How? Instructions for how to use the procedure are provided.
Why? The speech-language pathologist is interested in whether the child with tracheostomy is achieving an important milestone for all children, the establishment of canonical babbling (Oller & Eilers, 1988). Speaking children who are tracheostomized or recently decannulated are slow to use consonants and slow to achieve the .2 ratio of canonical syllables to utterances established by Oller and Eilers as the criterion for achieving canonical babbling (Bleile, 1998).

Research Support

Bleile (1998) documented the percentage of canonical syllables used by two children who had been recently decannulated. One child reported by Locke and Pearson (1990) exhibited 2% canonical syllables 1 month after decannulation, at 21 months. The other child studied by Bleile and colleagues exhibited 6% canonical syllables at approximately 32 months, 6 weeks after decannulation (Bleile, Stark, & Silverman McGowan, 1993). Typically, infants will exhibit 20% canonical syllables between 6 to 9 months.

Procedures:

1. Base the calculation of percentage of canonical syllables on a sample of a minimum of 50 spontaneous utterances. An utterance is a single breath with no more than 1 second of internal silence in the breath.

2. Count the number of canonical syllables. An utterance may contain more than one. A canonical syllable is defined according to the following criteria:

   a. A vowel plus a consonant of normal duration and formant transition. The syllable is phonated normally and with normal pitch.

   b. Coughs, cries, sneezes and grunts are excluded from analysis.

   c. Syllables that contain a glottal stop or glottal fricative as the consonant are also excluded.

3. Count the number of spontaneous utterances.

4. Divide the number of canonical syllables by the number of utterances.

5. Children are thought to have reached the canonical babbling stage when they exhibit a ratio of .2 or greater of canonical syllables to utterances (or a percentage of 20%), which typically occurs from 6 to 9 months in children who are developing language normally (Oller & Eilers, 1988).
6. The procedures outlined here are based on those used by Oller and Eilers, 1988.

ASSESSING THE SYLLABLE STRUCTURE LEVEL

Who? The child with tracheostomy who has been vocalizing for several months with a speaking valve and is capable of complex productions or the child who was recently decannulated and is capable of producing multiple syllables.
What? A procedure for assessing the syllable structure complexity of the child's utterances.
When? The speech-language pathologist would use this procedure when he/she wished to show the changes in complexity of syllable use. The procedure would be appropriate for use with a child who was just placed with a speaking valve or just decannulated, and the speech-language pathologist wished to document developmental changes in syllable structure use.
Where? May be employed at home or in the hospital where the child is comfortable vocalizing.
How? Instructions for how to use the procedure are provided.
Why? The speech-language pathologist is interested in whether the child with tracheostomy is making progress by increasing the length and complexity of utterances. An increase in the syllable structure level may indicate that the child is gaining motor or respiratory control and is able to articulate longer and/or more complex syllables in a single breath.

Research Support

Paul and Jennings (1992) showed that children who are developing language normally, generally, exhibited an average syllable structure level of greater than 2 by 24 months of age. Late talkers were shown by these researchers to exhibit syllable structures at levels 1 and 2, but few syllables at Level 3. Keep in mind that children with tracheostomies may not have had numerous opportunities to vocalize, and they may not have the breath support with the tracheostomy in place to support complex syllables of Levels 2 and 3.

Procedures and Instructions

Rate 20 to 50 child vocalizations and place them in one of the following three categories. When all the ratings are completed, add all the ratings that have been assigned (1, 2, or 3). Divide the sum of the ratings by the number of vocalizations included in the ratings.

Categories of Syllable Structure:

LEVEL 1:

Vocalization consists of a voiced vowel, voiced syllabic consonant [l] or a consonant + vowel (CV) containing a glottal stop or glide [wa] as the consonant.

LEVEL 2:

Vocalization consists of a vowel + consonant [VC] or consonant + vowel + consonant [CVC] with the same consonant initially and finally (voicing differences in the CVC are disregarded) or CV with consonants other than those in Level 1.

LEVEL 3:

Vocalizations consist of syllables with two or more different consonants, voicing differences in the consonants are disregarded. For example, [dati] is rated a Level 2 utterance, while [pati] is rated a Level 3 utterance. (Paul and Jennings, 1992; Paul, 1995).

DECISION MAKING IN SELECTING AN APPROPRIATE COMMUNICATION SYSTEM

Who? The child with tracheostomy who is likely to be cannulated over a period of one year or longer and will require ongoing assessment of the most effective and efficient communication system(s), based on his/her abilities.
What? Decision making regarding communication systems, based on assessment of communication and areas supporting communication.
When? When the speech-language pathologist and family have questions about the most appropriate communication system(s) for the child.
Where? In a comfortable room in the home or clinic.
How? Set up an assessment that incorporates the questions and issues outlined below.
Why? The child with long-term tracheostomy may be at risk for long-term speech and/or language difficulties; therefore appropriate systems that help to reduce frustration and provide the child with a means to communicate are crucial to helping reduce the potential risk of speech and language delay (Silverman McGowan, Bleile, Fus, & Barnas, 1993). It is also important to establish if the child is communicating for a variety of reasons.

Establishing a System for Immediate Use

Assessing a child's ability to use a verbal versus a nonverbal communication system is not easy. Many families and speech-language pathologists may elect to have a child use several systems at a time. A number of considerations will determine how the communication systems evolve over time. A primary consideration is the availability of a system that the child can use immediately and that is also compatible with the child's current communication and associated developmental skills. For example, a gesture or sign system may be used for the very young child (child 4–12 months) with tracheostomy who has been recently tracheostomized and for whom production of audible vocalizations are not realistic at the present time. An immediate system permits the child to communicate, thereby reducing frustration. The immediate system of signing may also serve the role of permitting the child to convey concepts that other children can easily convey, but the child with tracheostomy would not be able to communicate through words for some time. The same child may be a future candidate for a speaking valve based on his/her medical status. In the meantime, the speech-language pathologist may work with the family to facilitate the future use of a verbal system for this child. See Box 2–6 for an example of a communication program that affords a child an immediate communication program while improving language skills for use with future communication systems.

BOX 2–6. Establishing a Communication System for Immediate Use, Improving Language and Overall Development, and Planning for Future Communication Systems

Client:

Ben, age 12 months, exhibited an omphalocele at birth that required surgery, long-term ventilation and tracheostomy. He was hospitalized for 10 months. Ben shows near-age-level cognitive and receptive language skills. He is not vocalizing currently. Ben's omphalocele and ventilator restrict his motor movements, but he sits unsupported and is beginning to crawl. For the past 4 months he has been learning signs and his parents and visiting nurse sign with him. Ben was evaluated for a speaking valve, but gastroesophageal reflux prohibits placement currently.

Communication Goals and Treatment Program:

1. Improve receptive vocabulary for common people, objects, and events in his environment (maintain age-level-appropriate receptive skills as a foundation for expressive skills if Ben is eligible for a speaking valve).
2. Train Ben and important people in his home in signs for people, objects, and events Ben understands.
3. Encourage exploration of toys while seated in high chair and while on a blanket on floor to encourage movement (place interesting object just out of reach to encourage signing for the object).
4. Encourage turn-taking with parents through nonverbal means—exchange of smiles, hand movements, exchanging or pushing objects back and forth, exchanging noises or squeals.
5. Have parents attempt to occlude stoma for brief periods to encourage sound production and during imitative, turn-taking exchanges (help to acclimate Ben to feeling of using upper airway).
6. Reevaluate reflux within 1 month. Consult with occupational therapist about positioning to reduce reflux. Consult with nutritionist about food intake (amount, types) to reduce reflux.

Providing a System That Affords Flexibility

Along with the establishment of an immediate means of communication, the speech-language pathologist will want to select a communication system(s) that will meet the child's communication needs over a longer period of time. Considerations in selecting a particular system may include: (a) the amount of time needed to train the child and family in using the system, (b) the developmental demands placed on the child when using the system, and (c) the ease with which the family can understand and use the system. A system that requires some work on the part of the child and the speech-language pathologist is warranted if it is the best long-term option for a child.

In summary, the considerations in selecting a communication system should include: (a) ability of the system to provide a means of communication and to reduce the child's frustration, (b) ability of a system to allow a child to express concepts not otherwise expressed, (c) ability of a system to permit reciprocal interaction, (d) selection of a system according to a realistic evaluation of child's cognitive and motor abilities that support the child's use of the system with ease, (e) a decision based on balancing the time invested in training or setting up system with the length of time child will use the system.

SELECTING AN APPROPRIATE COMMUNICATION SYSTEM FOR EACH CHILD

Box 2–7 outlines some of the major decision points and factors to consider in making decisions about an appropriate communication system for each child and his/her family.

Making an informed decision will involve assessing not only the child's communication skills, but also the child's motor and cognitive abilities. The child's medical status and the medical condition that necessitated the tracheostomy will also strongly affect the type of communication system chosen for each child. Important questions to be asked or issues to be addressed in the developmental areas supporting communication are outlined below.

Assessment of Areas Supporting Communication

The speech-language pathologist will want to conduct an assessment in the areas outlined in Box 2–7, using measures with which he/she is familiar and that are appropriate to the child's level of functioning (See Table 2–8). Questions to be addressed rather than specific measures will also be presented.

BOX 2–7. Options and Associated Skills in the Selection of a Communication System for Children with Tracheostomies

Option 1:

Child vocalizes with stoma occluded

Prerequisite Skills or Conditions:

Child is able to produce sound, but the medical status does not support immediate use of speaking valve

Option 2:

Child vocalizes with speaking valve, electrolarynx, or esophageal speech*

Prerequisite Skills or Conditions:

Child is able to produce sound. Medical and respiratory status support the use of a speaking valve

Long-term system is desired.
Training is needed for child to use longer utterances

* Use of an electrolarynx or esophageal speech will also afford children opportunities to practice vocalizing. An electrolarynx provides an immediate system for vocal practice with some training. Esophageal speech will require considerable training. The vocal quality of either option may not be acceptable to some families.

Option 3:

Child uses gestures

Prerequisite Skills or Conditions:

Child is unable to produce sound
Child shows appropriate motor skills and receptive language skills to gesture
Immediate system is desired

Option 4:

Child uses signs

Prerequisite Skills or Conditions:

Child may or may not be able to produce sound, but cannot produce words
Child recognizes symbols
Child has manual dexterity to sign (ability to bring hands to midline and more dexterity required than for gesture use)
Immediate use of a limited set of symbols is afforded
Training is needed for child to use strings of signs

Option 5:

Child uses augmentative system (picture board, electronic board) to communicate

Prerequisite Skills or Conditions:

Child shows sufficient motor dexterity to point to or select items; child supports head and trunk to see and make selections

Cognitive skills support picture-referent correspondence or symbol or letter recognition

Long-term system is desired

Medical Status-Issues and Questions:

A determination of the child's medical status and candidacy for a speaking valve or for removal of the tracheal tube or ventilator support will be the most likely starting point in the assessment process.

- ❖ Is the child's health likely to stabilize and to permit periods of alertness in which parents and professionals can initiate observation of communication behaviors?
- ❖ What procedures need to be followed by parents and professionals so as not to compromise the child's respiration? What level of activities are permitted at the present time?
- ❖ Will the child require long-term ventilation in addition to the tracheostomy? Will the type of ventilator interfere with or aid the child's ability to vocalize?
- ❖ Does the child's medical condition support the eventual use of a speaking valve?
- ❖ If the child has a medical condition for which use of a speaking valve is contraindicated, is the condition likely to resolve in the future (gastrointestinal reflux)? Will surgery be required to resolve the contraindications (type of obstruction)?

INSTRUCTIONS:

Many of these questions will be addressed by a team of developmental and medical specialists. For the child who is hospitalized, the otolaryngologist, respiratory therapist, speech-language pathologist, occupational therapist, physical therapist, nursing staff, and parents will discuss the child's symptoms and progress. The speech-language pathologist will do a careful review of each child's medical chart. The presence of vocal paralysis, tracheal or subglottic stenosis, excessive granulation tissue, and tracheomalacia or fistula are typical contraindications to use of a speaking valve. However, the speech-language pathologist will consult with the otolaryngologist and the child's pediatrician because the presence of one of these conditions does not automatically rule out use of a speaking valve. If the granulation or stenosis is not severe, the child may still be eligible for a speaking valve, and the otolaryngologist will make the determination of candidacy. If the child is at home, he/she is followed on a regular basis through outpatient clinics (seen by a minimum team of medical staff, speech-language pathologist, and respiratory therapist) at the hospital where he/she was originally treated or by the otolaryngologist or pulmonologist who completed the tracheostomy.

Motor and Cognitive Skills: Issues and Questions/Relating Gross and Fine Motor Skills to Speaking and Feeding Skills

USE OF A GESTURE SYSTEM:

- ❖ Does the child sit upright with support of a chair or bolster?
- ❖ Does the child extend his/her arm to reach for objects?
- ❖ Does the child imitate an adult's gestures?
- ❖ Does the child indicate his/her needs by pointing?

Instructions: The speech-language pathologist and occupational therapist, along with the developmental specialist or physical therapist, will note the child's fine and gross motor development in relation to the development of communication and feeding skills (See Table 2–14). Although the child with tracheostomy may be slow to develop some skills, the child will likely progress through a normal sequence. The professional team and the parents will plan for a communication system based on the child's current level of functioning and ability to support a communication system, and the rate of development. If a child is making good progress in motor development and not does not currently exhibit skills for particular systems, the professional team will try to anticipate if the child will be a future candidate for a system, based on the degree of progress shown.

USE OF A SIGN SYSTEM:

- ❖ Does the child imitate a sequence of gestures?
- ❖ Does the child bring his/her hands to midline?
- ❖ Does the child imitate hand and/or finger configurations?

USE OF A COMMUNICATION BOARD:

- ❖ Does the child sit upright with support?
- ❖ Does the child indicate items with eyes or head or point with hand or finger?
- ❖ Does the child have appropriate vision to see pictures and cognition skills to recognize pictures?
- ❖ Does the child exhibit symbol-to-meaning correspondence (recognizes that a symbol or picture refers to the real world object or event)?

TABLE 2–14. Development of Gross Motor, Fine Motor, Speech Production, and Feeding Skills from Birth to 15 Months of Age

Age/ Months	*Gross Motor*	*Fine Motor*	*Speech Production*	*Feeding*
Birth	Moro, palmar grasp, tonic brynthine reflexes are prominent	Shoulders mildly retracted Hands frequently closed	Uses nasalized vowels Starting closure of back of vocal tract	Gentle support of head and extremities needed for feeding
	Turns heads from side to side in supine position			
	Head lags on pull to sit			
3–4	Primitive reflexes less prominent Increased midline head position in supine position	Hands open Midline hand play	Velar consonants and front or central vowels are prominent Varies jaw position for vowels	Suckle and rooting reflex less prominent Hands frequently in mouth
	Head in line with trunk while sitting			Less head, trunk support needed
				Spoon feeding begins
6–7	Absence of primitive reflexes	Unilateral reach and grasp	Tongue lateralization (7 mos.)	Suckle and rooting reflexes diminish
	Anterior and lateral propping reactions	Objects to mouth	Up and down movement of jaw	Munching appears Holds bottle Reaches for food
	Brief independent sitting		Larger oral cavity with growth of mandible Tongue tip sounds (6 mos.)	Sits supported in high chair
9–10	Sits steady for 10–15 minutes	Immature pincer grasp	Jaw separate from oral movement during biting	Increased independent sitting for feeding
	Stands holding onto person or furniture	Reaches and leans forward, then recovers balance	Control over opening and closing of vocal tract Precise stops by 9 mos. Fricatives (f, v, th, sh, s, z)	Finger feeding
12–15	Walks independently	Diminished mouthing of objects Picks up and releases objects	Lips active in chewing Vertical and diagonal jaw movement	Throws food Holds cup Uses spoon
		Spontaneous supination of hands	Full range of vowels and consonants used	
		Grasps and manipulates long slender objects	Imitates speech sounds	

Note. Adapted from Rogers, B. T. (1996). Neurodevelopmental presentation of dysphagia pp. 274. *Seminars in Speech and Language, 17* (4), pp. 269–281. Reprinted with permission of Thieme Medical Publishers, New York.

Instructions/Cognitive and Motor Support Needed for Various Communication Systems: A thorough evaluation of a child's cognitive and motor skills are essential for selecting and establishing an effective communication system. Cognitive and motor skills can be be assessed through a combination of the following methods: (a) informal observations, (b) use of checklists, (c) feedback from other professionals and family,

(d) trial use of various communication systems and, (e) administration of standardized measures. Generally, many children can learn a signed vocabulary if they display the ability to position themselves to view people and objects in their environment and if they display basic imitation of gestures and knowledge of common concepts commensurate with developmental skills of 6–12 months. Use of communication boards will likely require more advanced cognitive skills. For example, the recognition of pictures is generally an 18-month cognitive skill. Table 2–15 outlines some of the cognitive and motor skills needed to successfully use several communication systems and the approximate ages at which these skills are acquired. Comprehensive assessment for the child with tracheostomy involves a keen knowledge of early development and an ability to integrate information from various developmental areas in developing an intervention plan.

TABLE 2–15. Cognitive and Motor Support Required for Various Communication Systems

System	*Skills*	*Approximate Age Skill Acquired*
Occlusion of Stoma	Fine motor control to bring hands to midline	Bring hands to midline, 4–6 months
	Ability to follow simple directions	15 months, 12–15 months if context provided
Use of Electrolarynx	Fine motor control to operate on/off switch	18–24 months, ability to twist wrist and to hold and place objects (cup)
	Fine motor control and strength to hold device at throat	24 months, ability to hold and use hammer
Use of Manual Signs	Ability to imitate motor actions	9–12 months, some simple signs at 6–9 months
	Ability to match sign with referent	12 months, ability to imitate deferred action (hold representation)
Alternative Communication	Cognitive ability to match symbol to its referent	Recognizes pictures, 12–15 months
Picture Pointing Board	Gross motor ability to indicate by pointing	Pointing, 12–14 months

SECTION 3

INTERVENTION FOR THE CHILD 0–3 YEARS DURING AND AFTER TRACHEOSTOMY

INTERVENTION WHILE THE TRACHEOSTOMY IS IN PLACE

This section will focus on intervention strategies that the speech-language pathologist can use while a child is tracheostomized, for the purpose of stimulating speech and language development along with general development (cognitive, social and oral-motor skills). The speech-language pathologist is faced with a two-tiered decision in intervention planning, which involves answering the following questions:

1. What is(are) the best possible communication system(s) to facilitate speech and language development for this child?
2. What intervention goals (what content areas) will promote speech and language development in this child?

Issues that the speech-language pathologist might consider in determining an answer to the first question were reviewed in Section 2. Section 3 will provide information to help the speech-language pathologist in answering the second question.

Particular intervention goals that will likely serve the needs of many children while they have a tracheostomy in place have been selected based on the speech and language limitations of children with tracheostomies cited in the literature. Specific guidelines for carrying out the specific goals come from intervention procedures conducted with other populations who have also experienced speech and language difficulties due to early environments that are less than optimal for learning language (children with cerebral palsy, medically fragile infants).

The *content* of intervention will be the focus of this chapter. Selected goals based on research findings for children with a tracheostomies in place or for infants who are at risk will be reviewed and include the following:

1. Modification of the early environment of infants in the intensive care unit and training in behavioral strategies to promote increased ability of the infant to attend to stimuli and interact with caregivers (both are important to later language development).
2. The improvement of communication signals, either verbal or nonverbal (Yoder & Feagans, 1988), and incorporation of early communication into social routines (Warren & Yoder, 1998).
3. The improvement of communication for a variety of functions, including regulating the behavior of others, being social, and establishing joint attention, through verbal or nonverbal means (Warren & Yoder, 1998).
4. Stimulation of early cognitive skills. Training of the functional use of objects and/or exposure to a variety of objects, actions and events about which children can communicate through verbal or nonverbal means (Olswang & Pinder, 1995).
5. Normalization of early oral-motor experiences and stimulating oral-motor skills with the goal of improving oral motor functions needed for speech development.
6. Establishment of opportunities to vocalize and stimulation of vocalizations (Morrison, 1998). Opportunities to vocalize may not be currently available to the child for medical reasons (e.g., the speech-language pathologist serves as an advocate for the child and family to negotiate various oral communication options for the child). This section will also highlight specific issues the speech-language pathologist needs to be aware of when matching a tracheostomy tube/ventilator and speaking device to the child's respiratory and anatomical abilities and restrictions.

From the research literature, a pattern of speech and language characteristics exhibited by children with long-term tracheostomies is starting to emerge. The child with tracheostomy is at risk for speech as well as language difficulties. These risks may arise from insults to neurological function or from multiple disruptions to the early language learning environment. The research findings suggest that:

1. Receptive language as well as expressive language can be affected in children who undergo long-term tracheostomies, with expressive language being more involved than receptive language (Kaslon & Stein, 1985; Morrison, 1998; Simon, Fowler & Handler, 1983).
2. Speech production difficulties can occur in children with long-term tracheostomies including vowel production, phonological and/or oral-motor difficulties (Kamen & Watson, 1991; Kertoy et al., 1999).
3. The few longitudinal investigations of children with tracheostomies that exist suggest that children rebound in expressive language skills following decannulation, but the recovery is slow (Locke & Pearson, 1990; Bleile, 1998). Some children may take several years for expressive language skills to match age and/or cognitive expectations. The biggest obstacle for these children appears to be the poor speech production skills that result from long periods with little or no vocal practice (Bleile, 1998). Even after expressive language skills improve, the child may experience subtle speech production difficulties.
4. Those children with tracheostomies who also exhibit complicated medical histories and neurological involvement are at considerable risk for speech and language difficulties (Arvedson & Brodsky, 1992; Gallagher & Watkin, 1998).

Research support for selecting the guidelines and procedures that accompany the goals is based primarily on research work completed with children with phonological delays and children with restrictions on language learning resulting from lack of hearing or poor mobility. The few intervention programs that have been conducted with children with tracheostomies are cited, along with developmental information and intervention procedures for children who have been restricted in their early language use or who have experienced early deprivation in exploring their environments.

FORMAT FOR PRESENTING INTERVENTION PROCEDURES

For each procedure reviewed in this section, answers to the following questions will be provided along with the research literature that supports the use of the procedure or provides information about the language performance of children utilizing the procedure.

Who? Indicates the age and/or developmental and health status of the child for whom the procedure is most appropriate.
What? Indicates the subject or topic of the procedure.
When? Indicates the circumstances under which the parent or speech-language pathologist might find using the procedure most helpful.
Where? Indicates the physical location or the condition of the child to optimally complete the procedure.
How? Indicates the general instructions for completing the procedure. Specific instructions are frequently provided in a separate paragraph.
Why? Indicates the importance of the topic or procedure for children with tracheostomies and their families.

Research Support

Provides a rationale for the topic or use of a particular procedure. Specific research findings are included.

PROVIDING ENVIRONMENTAL MODIFICATIONS AND BEHAVIORAL STRATEGIES

Children with bronchopulmonary dysplasia or other complicated medical conditions that require tracheostomies and hospitalization will benefit from modifications to the NICU environment that reduce the amount of light and noise, and the number of people. The modifications also include management of the timing and clustering of daily care activities. Box 3–1 outlines the Minimal Handling Protocol (VandenBerg & Franck, 1990). This protocol is part of the developmental care recommended for children with bronchopulmonary dysplasia and forms the foundation of developmental stimulation for medically fragile children. The protocol would be carried out by all staff on the NICU according to the guidelines developed in a particular unit. The procedures would also be conducted by the speech-language pathologist, the physical therapist, or any other professional. They will take place prior to delivering developmental stimulation to facilitate the child's readiness for programming.

Environmental modifications should not be viewed as a program carried out by professionals in which the child plays a passive role. The modifications are initially enacted to help the child preserve energy, reduce agitation, and gain weight (VandenBerg & Franck, 1990). A major part of the protocol is also to handle and position the child to encourage self-regulation on the part of the child (Creger, 1989). For example, placing a child in a side-lying position and helping to bring his/her hand to the mouth for him/her to suck calms the child. As the child grows and improves his/her behavioral organization, he/she is able to respond more appropriately to environmental stimuli without excessive expenditure of energy and able to regulate himself/herself more efficiently (holding on to mother's finger, sucking on a finger).

HELPING THE INFANT RESPOND TO THE ENVIRONMENT

BOX 3–1. Minimal Handling Protocol

Protect from Light
- Shade infant's eyes (with blanket)
- Cover incubator or crib with blanket

Protect from Noise
- Give reports about patients away from crib
- Eliminate phones ringing
- Cushion trash receptacles
- Close incubator doors gently
- Remove noise sources
- Avoid tearing paper near infant

(continues)

BOX 3–1. *(continued)*

Protect from Overstimulation
- Cluster nursing care activities
- Allow 2–3-hour periods of undisturbed sleep
- No routine postural drainage or suctioning
- Contain limbs during suctioning

Provide Boundaries
- Position prone or side lying
- Cover/wrap/swaddle
- Use blanket rolls to tuck around infant (sides, head, feet)
- Provide objects the infant can suck or grasp

Note. Adapted from Vandenberg, K. A. and Franck, L. S. (1990). Behavioral issues for infants with BPD. In C. Lund (Ed.), *BPD: Building strategies for total patient care*, pp. 114–152. Santa Rosa, CA: NICU, Inc. Reprinted with permission of NICU, Inc., Santa Rosa, CA.

Who? Medically fragile infants in the NICU.
What? Behavioral strategies for the infant with bronchopulmonary dysplasia/other chronic medical conditions.
When? To be incorporated as much as possible into each child's daily schedule.
Where? NICU or pediatric critical care unit.
How? The general procedures outlined below should be modified to meet the needs of individual children.
Why? Reducing the amount and intensity of environmental stimuli allows the child to organize his/her behavior and to regulate herself/himself in response to the environment. With reduced stress and agitation and with strategies to allow them to gain greater control, medically fragile infants gain weight and are hospitalized for shorter periods (Als, 1997). The environmental modifications become a part of the early developmental program for medically fragile infants. Once the child begins to respond to his/her environment without excessive expenditure of energy (rapid respiration and heart rate), oral-motor and feeding, cognitive, and parent-child interaction and communication activities are overlayed on the environmental modifications.

Research Support

The outcome of employing behavioral strategies and environmental modifications for children with tracheostomies has not been studied. However, a large percentage of children have tracheostomies as a result of bronchopulmonary dysplasia or respiratory distress (percentages vary from 26% to 69%)(Arcand & Granger, 1988; Wood & Singer, 1990; Singer, Wood & Lambert, 1985). Clearly, children with tracheostomies are treated with developmental programming in NICUs along with other children with complex medical conditions. Table 3–1 reviews strategies for working with children with bronchopulmonary dysplasia.

TABLE 3–1. Behavioral Strategies for Fragile Infants with BPD

Strategies	*Goals or Examples*
Environmental protection	Reduce noise & lights, and reduce lights to create night/day cycle
Handling	Avoid abrupt movements
	Use touch gently and efficiently
Positioning	Position the infant in a flexed or side-lying position to encourage flexion
	Use blankets, bolsters to maintain flexion
Soothing	Reduce activity
	Cover or encourage sucking on the child's hand
Promoting interactions	Reduce noise and light
	Use a screen for privacy
	Provide support to encourage alertness (hand in infant's hand or on chest)
	Attempt to talk or look at infant as he/she will tolerate
	Encourage attending for longer periods
Gavage feeding	Time feeding with sleep cycle
	Reduce light and noise
	Avoid social interaction
	Position side lying or hold if not overstimulating to infant
	Provide pacifier to suck
Making the crib a learning environment	Increase alertness and visual attention
	Use a mirror to encourage gazing
	Use one toy to encourage attending
	Encourage fine motor skills
	Place rattle in the child's hand to encourage reaching and grasping as well as visual attending

Note. Adapted from Vandenberg, K. A. and Franck, L. S. (1990). Behavioral issues for infants with BPD. In C. Lund (Ed.), *BPD: Building strategies for total patient care*, pp. 114–152. Santa Rosa, CA: NICU, Inc. Reprinted with permission of NICU, Inc., Santa Rosa, CA.

Procedures

Infants with bronchopulmonary dysplasia benefit from careful timing of caregiving and intervention. The following procedures describe the sequence of care prior to, during, and following intervention to ensure that the infant is not overstimulated.

Prior to Intervention

Approach the infant and observe the child for a specified period of time (3–5 minutes, most NICUs will have an established procedure).

During care

1. Observe the infant for signs of stress during care.
2. Conduct care with smooth movements.
3. Limit the number of stimuli presented at a time (don't talk while feeding the child).

4. Provide containment or physical support during care.
5. Set up screens for privacy and noise reduction if possible.

Following care

1. Gradually remove touch.
2. Soothe the child to promote efficient recovery.
3. Observe the child for 3–5 minutes to note the time needed to recover. (Time to settle following care should decrease gradually; note techniques that help to soothe, and apply these each time.)

ORAL STIMULATION AND NONNUTRITIVE SUCKING PROCEDURES

Children with tracheostomies due to airway obstructions, neuromuscular problems, or respiratory distress are at risk for oral-motor and feeding difficulties (Arvedson & Brodsky, 1993; Harris, 1986). Some of these children will be fed by tube for a period of time, and oral stimulation may help to simulate normal oral-motor experiences. The procedures presented here are general guidelines. Each child's tolerance of touch, his/her neurobehavioral organization, and his/her readiness for oral stimulation should be carefully evaluated by the multidisciplinary developmental team (speech-language pathologist, occupational therapist, physiotherapist, pediatrician or neonatologist, nurse specialist). An individualized program is then prepared for each child. The information presented here will guide the speech-language pathologist in developing appropriate programs.

STIMULATING NONNUTRITIVE SUCKING

Who?	Children with tracheostomies beginning in infancy who are tube fed or who are fed orally and require oral-motor experiences. Children with obstructions at or above the larynx are likely to require tube feeding, as will children with neurological conditions that hinder cough or gag, or result in insufficient muscular strength, preventing feeding.
What?	Procedures for Stimulation of Nonnutritive Sucking.
When?	Procedures can be incorporated into tube feeding routine for those infants being fed by tube so that they gain some oral-motor experience. Procedures can also be used when children are making the transition to oral feedings. Children who are oral feeders, but who experience weak or uncoordinated suck, may also benefit.
Where?	In the NICU, hospital or home by trained professionals and by parents following demonstration/training with the procedures.
How?	Specific suggestions to follow will be outlined.
Why?	Most occupational therapists and speech-language pathologists begin oral stimulation activities early for children who are at risk for feeding and speech difficulties. The clinical procedures are conducted to provide the infant/child with normal oral-motor experiences.

Research Support

Pinelli and Symington (2000) reviewed the literature on the therapeutic effects of nonnutritive sucking (NNS). The results of the impact of NNS on physiological (heart rate), behavioral organization (fussiness), and feeding related behaviors (intestinal transit time, time to establish nipple feeding, etc.) were reviewed from 19 research studies. Pinelli and Symington (2000) found that there were mixed results regarding the impact of NNS on the following long-term variables: weight gain, energy intake, heart rate, oxygen saturation, intestinal transit time, and age at full oral feeding. The studies reviewed showed short-term, clinical gains for children in the experimental versus control groups: shorter time to establish nipple feeding, decrease in time infant spent in fussy or awake states, an increase in the speed with which the infant settled after feedings, a decrease in the defensive behaviors shown while feeding. Further investigation of the long-term benefits of NNS was recommended by these authors. Table 3–2 reviews procedures for stimulating nonnutritive sucking.

TABLE 3–2. Procedures to Stimulate Nonnutritive Sucking

Procedure	*When Used*	*How Used*
Stroking face	Initial approach with oral hypersensitivity	Palm of hand or finger rhythmically from periphery to mouth; firm, but gentle strokes
Stroking tongue	Infants lacking consistent sucking rhythm	Place fingertip at midtongue; stroke toward front of tongue with pressure down on tongue 4 to 6 times; use a rate of 1 stroke/second for NS and rate of 2 strokes/second for NNS; pause, then repeat after several seconds
Pacifier or finger	Infants with mild sucking incoordination Infants with reduced cheek tone	Pacifier or finger is placed in mouth and held in place if infant attempts to push it out
Cotton swab dipped in water, formula, or breast milk	Infants lacking coordinated suck/swallow/breathe sequence; child is not ready for oral intake of liquids, but taste experience is desired	Swab is placed at midtongue with downward pressure to release minimal amount of liquid; stroke as with little finger; repeat as tolerated in pleasurable way
Reduce sensory stimulation	Lack of ability to integrate competing sensations	Reduce noise and light levels Use rocking, walking, rhythmic music if tolerated Music should have regular rhythm Use containment

Note. From Arvedson, J. & Brodsky, L. (1993). Pediatric swallowing and feeding: Assessment and management. San Diego: Singular Publishing. Reprinted with permission of Singular Publishing Group, Inc.

Specific Instructions for Stroking Procedure

1. Start peripherally with palm or finger.
2. Begin at the ears and move centrally to cheek, chin, and mouth.
3. Use circular movements. (Arvedson & Brodsky, 1993)

Specific Instructions for Sucking Procedure

1. Place gloved finger on middle of tongue. Move from middle to front of tongue with downward pressure.
2. Stroke at the rate of 1 stroke per second for nutritive sucking and at 2 strokes per second for nonnutritive sucking, for 6 to 8 strokes.
3. Hold finger in the middle of tongue to approximate the nipple for several seconds to see if the child starts to suck.
4. Perform the procedure two times per day for 5–10 minutes per session when fed by tube or orally.
5. Monitor the child for signs of stress or fatigue.
6. Pair oral stimulation with your voice if the child will tolerate more than one stimulus at a time, in order to pair communication and feeding experiences (Arvedson & Brodsky, 1993).

Specific instructions to Provide Taste Experience (Initiate Swallow)

1. Vary tastes (very small amount of water, breast milk, juice) to initiate a swallow.
2. Place a small drop of liquid on a cotton swab and note if child swallows.
3. Use only small amounts so the rhythmic suck is maintained.
4. Very gradually increase the number of drops used (Arvedson and Brodsky, 1993).

GOALS FOR STIMULATING NORMAL ORAL-MOTOR EXPERIENCES

Who? Children with tracheostomies, beginning with infants. Children who are being fed by tube. Children for whom positive oral-motor experiences are a goal in order to facilitate oral feeding or speech or to improve oral sensation.
What? Oral-motor goals and activities for stimulating normal oral-motor experiences.
When? Starting in infancy and when goals are prescribed by occupational therapist and/or speech-language pathologist.
Where? Quiet area in the hospital or home.
How? See applications/examples provided.
Why? Children with tracheostomies are at risk for developing problems with oral-motor functioning or oral-motor sensitivity. This increased risk may be due to aversive experiences in the oral-motor region, or to the lack of normal movements that accompany oral feeding (if tube fed), or to retraction of the tongue when the child is positioned on his/her back consistently in the NICU.

Research Support

The following goals are routinely prescribed for children who are at risk for not developing normal oral-motor functioning, including children with tracheostomies (Driver, 2000) (Table 3–3). No research studies have documented the long-term effects of oral-motor stimulation on the development of speech or oral feeding in children with tracheostomies.

TABLE 3–3. Goals and Activities for Stimulating Normal Oral-Motor Experiences in Children with Tracheostomies

Goal	*Example of Suggested Actvity[a]*
Building a desire to use the mouth	Have the child touch his/her body and mouth, lips with own hand
Normalizing the response to oral stimuli	Have child explore objects with hands, mouth, tongue
	Use pacifiers with bright colors and bumpy surfaces to encourage the child's mouthing of toys; try to involve the tongue as well as gums in mouthing
	Play peek-a-boo with washcloth and place it gently at child's cheek and mouth as part of the activity
Improving control of the pharyngeal airway	Use a forward head position to reduce tongue retraction and increase diameter of airway
Using touch and movement communicatively	Combine sound or music in a playful way with touch or movement Examples: encourage louder or longer sounds while a child swings; make silly sounds while the child sucks on pacifier or mouths a teether; encourage sound use while tapping or rocking the child to sleep; use music to encourage rhythmical breathing and sucking; mother and child take turns tasting a teether or finger

Note. Adapted from Morris, S. & Klein, M. (1987). *Prefeeding Skills: A comprehensive resource for feeding development*. Tucson, AZ: Therapy Skill Builders. Reproduced by permission. All rights reserved.

a = The appropriateness of these activities will vary widely for children with tracheostomies. Activities should be undertaken based on specific goals prescribed by the developmental team for a given child.

STIMULATING COGNITIVE SKILLS

Who? The child with tracheostomy under 12 months of age who is hospitalized or at home.
What? Guidelines for stimulating cognitive skills.
When? Activities can be incorporated into an infant's daily schedule and conducted by the primary nurse or the parents.
Where? Create a learning environment in the infant's immediate surroundings in the hospital or at home.
How? Through the use of materials and interactions as well as through the education of parents and staff about the importance of stimulating cognitive skills.
Why? The hospital environment is not ideally suited for the stimulation of cognitive and other developmental skills. Therefore, it is important to stimulate the child's attending to people and objects and to help the child explore his/her environment.

Research Support

There are no studies that have evaluated the effectiveness of stimulating cognitive activities in children or the long-term cognitive or communication development of children with tracheostomies. Some children with tracheostomies (some studies indicate as high as 51% of children with tracheostomies) exhibit neurological problems (Singer, Kercsmar, Legris, Orlowski, Hill, & Doershuck, 1989). Other children, without known cognitive deficits, may benefit from cognitive activities that facilitate normal development. Box 3–2 and Table 3–4 review ways for stimulating cognitive skills in the hospital and at home.

BOX 3–2. Guidelines for Stimulating Cognitive Skills in the Hospital

1. Create a learning area in the infant's immediate environment through placement of carefully selected items to stimulate attending (VandenBerg & Franck, 1990).
2. The environment should afford opportunities for increasing attention to visual, tactile, and auditory stimuli (Billeaud, 1998).
3. The use of a few items that are effective in getting the child to respond is more appropriate than overuse of items or the use of large toys or toys that may startle the child.
4. Change the items so that the child's environment varies as much as possible.
5. Change the child's position; try bolsters to achieve some opportunities for the child to explore objects and support his/her forearms while on his/her tummy. Hold the child for brief periods, if possible, so he/she has a different view of his/her surroundings.

Suggestions for Items to Stimulate Attending to Various Types of Stimuli

Visual Stimulation—Place a mirror where the infant can easily gaze at himself/herself or place one brightly covered object that attracts the child's attention at close range (VandenBerg & Franck, 1990). Move the object to different locations at the side and above the child so that the child gradually has to turn his/her head or body to view the object. Dangling objects of interest to the child also encourages grasping and reaching (VandenBerg and Franck, 1990).

Auditory Stimulation—Tape the mother's or father's voice so that the child can hear a familiar, soothing voice (Billeaud, 1998). Experiment with the use of babbling as a stimulus or the use of nursery rhymes or calming music as a stimulus. Encourage family members and staff to talk to each infant when the child is calm and alert.

Tactile Stimulation—Introduce materials with different surfaces gradually (smooth—such as a sheepskin, rough—such as a washcloth). Try the hand, arm, or tummy to note where/if the child will tolerate touch.

TABLE 3–4. Guidelines for Stimulating Cognitive Skills at Home for the Child with Tracheostomy

1. Gather appropriate toys—Help the family with gathering some appropriate toys to encourage auditory, visual, and tactile stimulation. These can be common objects found in the home.
2. Change the toys frequently to match the child's interests and level of cognitive development—Explain the importance of having/using objects that provide changing and increasingly interesting stimulation to the parents. Describe how the objects change as the child's cognitive and motor skills progress. For example, at 4 months, babies are interested in things they can hold, while at 12 to 15 months, they are ready to explore, and enjoy finding objects nearby.
3. Incorporate stimulation activities into everyday routines to increase the ease with which they can be completed—Help families with ways to incorporate exploration of toys or visual or auditory stimulation activities into everyday routines. For example, encourage the mother to provide the the child with a wooden spoon and a nonbreakable bowl to bang while she prepares a meal in the kitchen (6-month activity).
4. Follow the developmental chart provided to help in the selection of toys and activities.

Child's Developmental Age	*Appropriate Toys/Materials[a]*	*Skill Development*
4 months	Things to grasp	Tries to hold objects
	Bouncing on lap/provide support	Focuses on objects that are close or at a distance
6 months	Things to bang (spoon and bowl)	Puts objects in mouth
	Bath things	Transfers objects from one hand to the other
	Bouncer or swing	Bounces when held upright

(continues)

TABLE 3–4. *(continued)*

8 months	Crawling, moving around activities	Crawling begins
	Unbreakable mirror	Recognizes faces
	Finger puppets	Begins to understand words
	Picture books	
	Songs with rhymes, actions	
9 months	Small things to pick up	Gains control over individual fingers
		Reaches for toys when seated
	Dropping and picking up objects	Searches for toys dropped out of sight/hidden while child watches
12–15 months	Play telephone	Imitates and uses words
	Containers to fill and empty	Holds two objects in one hand
	Hide-and-find games	Remembers where objects belong
	Picture books	Recognizes objects in books, turns pages
15–18 months	Dance music	Balances and moves on feet
	Balls	Throws objects
	Paper and pencil	Makes side-to-side marks on paper
	Blocks	Builds a block tower
	Container with shaped objects	Fits shapes in holes
18–24 months	Dolls	Imitates actions with objects
	Dress up clothes	Plays make believe
	Dust, sweep, dig with mom and dad	Imitates actions with objects in context
	Photo album	Recognizes familiar faces
	Books with multiple, similar items	Matches identical objects

Note. Reproduced from *Entertaining and educating your preschool child* by permission of Usborne Publishing, 83-85 Saffron Hill, London ECIN 8RT, UK. Copyright Usborne Publishing Ltd. © 1993.

a = some materials may be appropriate for teaching multiple skills.

IMPROVING A CHILD'S USE OF SIGNALS

Who? Child with tracheostomy who is limited in communicating.
What? Procedures that can be used to shape a child's signals for communication and to increase the use of signals.
When? When the child with tracheostomy exhibits an awareness of his/her surroundings and is beginning to respond to social cues.
Where? In the home or hospital by parents or the speech-language pathologist.
How? Specific procedures will be outlined.
Why? The use of signals is the beginning of preverbal communication. All other communication follows from the child's initial responses to his/her environment and his/her ability to show an interest in people and objects. Children with communication delays frequently use signals that are difficult to interpret, and this may hinder the amount of parent-child interaction that occurs (Yoder, 1987).

Research Support

Two issues emerge from the literature about the use of signals by infants who have difficulties communicating. The number of initiations by a child and an increase in clarity of a child's signals both appear to be important to later language development. Snow (1989) showed that the number of initiations by children at 14 months was related to the size of their vocabularies at 20 months. Likewise, Wetherby, Yonclas, and Bryan (1989) determined that the rate at which children communicated (number of acts per minute) might be a useful indication of a child's later use of intentional communicative acts. In addition, Yoder and Feagans (1988) showed that mothers of children with more severe disabilities interpreted as many of a child's cues as communicative as did mothers of children with less severe disabilities. The important issue appeared to be the mother's ability to gradually and differentially respond to more conventional over less clear cues of the child.

Procedures and Guidelines:

The following guidelines will help parents and professionals to shape behaviors of children into early communication signals and turns.

Observe

1. Observe any signals the child is currently using (smiling, using gestures) (See Tables 2–7 and 2–9, in Assessment section).

   a. Note the context(s) in which the signals occur.

   b. Note how easy/difficult it is to interpret what the child is communicating through the signal.

Respond

1. Respond to signals that are communicative (e.g., smiling, turning head to familiar people, gesturing, signaling toward objects).
2. Respond by verbalizing or by drawing closer to the child or by giving the child the desired object.
3. See if the child will continue the behavior or maintain the interaction.
4. If the signal is not easily interpretable, begin to shape the signal into a behavior that serves a communicative purpose.

Shape

1. The child should signal toward a person(s) initially. For example, expect the child to acknowledge family members upon first entry to a room.
2. Later, the child will signal toward objects or events in his/her environment. (Pinder & Olswang, 1995).
Example:
If a child normally waves his hand toward an object to indicate his interest in the object, gradually expect a full hand point toward the object. Model pointing or reaching toward an object. Guide the child's hand the first few times in pointing. Once the child indicates with a clearer point, remove the physical prompt. Show more excitement when the full hand point is used than when other, less clear signals are used. Wait to give the child an object until the clearer signal is used.
3. If the child is slow to develop a pointing gesture, check to make sure the child has the motor and cognitive readiness for pointing (e.g., the child uses fingers individually and attends to objects consistently).

4. The speech-language pathologist will want to observe the child on an ongoing basis and help the family with determining clear and less clear signals and which signals should be encouraged.

GUIDELINES FOR ENCOURAGING TURN-TAKING BETWEEN PARENTS AND CHILD

Who? The child with tracheostomy who is responsive to his/her environment and is signaling, but who is communicating or interacting inconsistently.
What? Guidelines and procedures for encouraging turn-taking.
When? Frequently throughout the day when the child is alert and responsive to his/her environment.
Where? Home or hospital by parents or primary nurse.
How? Procedures are provided.
Why? The child's ability to imitate actions and to take turns is basic to establishing social routines. Within social routines, children learn intentional communication, attend to adult input, and gradually learn more complex play (Warren & Yoder, 1998).

Research Support

There are no research studies that have investigated the motor imitation and turn-taking of children with tracheostomies. Intervention procedures that focus on improving parent-child interaction have been shown to bring about changes in children's turn-taking as well as improvements in parents' strategies to get children to interact (Tannock & Girolametto, 1992).

Procedure for Encouraging Turn-taking

1. Notice and respond to what the child does (smiles, waves, looks at you, looks to object and reaches, hands toy to you, etc.).
2. Responding may take several forms. For the young child (4–8 months), imitate what the child does. Wait and see if the child will imitate you. If he/she doesn't do anything else, imitate the child's action and cue for another turn by looking, raising your eyebrows, and expecting more. For the child of 8 months or older, comment on what the child has done, and then cue the child to take another turn.
3. Taking turns can be the exchange of several looks in a row by the adult and child, the exchange of hand waves or claps or blowing kisses, or the exchange of funny noises.
4. Taking turns can also be incorporated into social routines. Social routines are turn-taking games such as peekaboo or daily rituals surrounding feeding, going to bed, etc.
5. Social routines may consist of a few turns or may be a song with a series of turns, actions, and words. Teaching the child routines helps him/her to anticipate what will come next. At first expect the child to experience the routine, then the child may come to understand some of the turns and actions. Finally, the child will anticipate when his/her turn has come or anticipate what will happen next (Manolson, 1992).

TEACHING THE FUNCTIONAL USE OF OBJECTS

Who? The child with tracheostomy in place who has had limited opportunities to manipulate and learn about objects and/or who is experiencing delays in receptive language.
What? Procedures that can be used to improve a child's knowledge of the functional use of objects.
When? A speech-language pathologist who is working with a child with tracheostomy in the hospital or who has been recently discharged from the hospital.
Where? In the home or the hospital by the speech-language pathologist with help from the parents.
How? Specific procedures will be outlined. (See Developmental Sequence in Table 3–5).
Why? Children with tracheostomies have limited opportunities to learn language while in the hospital. Some children with tracheostomies have exhibited delays in cognition or receptive language. One way to stimulate a child's understanding of his/her environment is through providing opportunities to mouth and handle objects to gradually understand how the objects are used in a functional way. Manipulation of objects is also related to the child's learning to gesture with objects (Bates, et al., 1989) and to use more complex play schemes (McCune,1995).

Research Support

Olswang and Pinder (1995) showed gains in the type of object play used by four children, ranging in age from 11.6 months to 13.6 months with cerebral palsy following a 12-week treatment program designed to train person-object looking. Three children, who primarily mouthed objects during baseline, moved to finger exploration with objects as well as showing and banging objects. One child who used fingers to explore objects at the start of the study moved to looking at and turning objects in different directions, along with banging objects. All children increased their knowledge of the types of actions that can be performed with different objects. Although no studies have investigated the outcome of training play with objects in children with tracheostomies, the findings of Olswang and Pinder (1995) may have implications for improving the object knowledge of children with tracheostomies.

General Guidelines:

Speech-language pathologists may want to refer to the developmental sequence provided in Table 3–5 for manipulating objects reviewed by Johnson-Martin, Jens, Attermeier, and Hacker (1991). The authors also provide specific procedures for helping to guide children along this developmental continuum.

TABLE 3–5. Developmental Sequence for Manipulating Objects

Age of Acquisition	*Activity*
3 months	Moves hand to mouth
3 months	Explores objects with mouth
6 months	Shakes, bangs toys placed in hand
6 months	Commonly performs four or more activities with objects
6 months	Explores objects and responds to their differences
9 months	Demonstrates appropriate activities with toys that have obviously different properties
9 months	Combines two objects in a functional manner

(continues)

TABLE 3–5. *(continued)*

12 months	Imitates activities related to the function of objects
15 months	Plays spontaneously with a variety of objects, demonstrating their functions (moving to symbolic use of objects)
18 months	Imitates adult behavior with props
21 months	Spontaneously engages in adult activities with props
24 months	Talks to dolls or animals and makes them interact with one another

Note. From Johnson-Martin, N. M., Jens, K. G., Attermeier, S. M. & Hacker, B. J. (1991). *The Carolina curriculum for infants and toddlers with special needs. Second Edition*. pp. 141–142. Reprinted with permission of Paul H. Brookes Publishing Co., Baltimore, MD.

Specific Procedures:

Based on several treatment outcomes prescribed by Olswang and Pinder (1995), the following goals and procedures may be used to improve the object knowledge of children with tracheostomies who have had limited opportunities to explore objects.

Provide a Time Each Day (If Possible) to Handle and Explore Objects

The time allowed may be as short as 10 minutes, but time for exploration should be provided. For children who are currently hospitalized, note times when the child is most alert. This may be when the family visits or it may be at 2 A.M., when the room is free from distractions. Designate a family member or member of the nursing staff to interact with the child. Also, provide a play box or basket with a variety of toys so that toys are readily available (See Table 3–6 for types of toys).

Present an Array of Toys

See what toys the child chooses and is attracted to. For children with physical limitations, place an object the child looks at within his/her hand or mouth. Guide the hand to mouth movement or the manipulation of the object with fingers as necessary. Name the object and talk about what the object does or comment on the child's actions with the object. Consider the best position—sitting in a chair with a tray of toys, sitting on the floor with toys around the child, positioned in a side-lying position or with arms over a bolster and on the tummy, to promote looking at and touching objects.

Encourage the child to manipulate the objects

Encourage the child to manipulate the objects that he/she chooses first. Gradually introduce different toys that vary in texture or function or number of movable parts.

Work Toward Goals

Work toward the following goals (refer to Table 3–6):

1. Increase the amount of overall time the child spends with objects and/or the time spent with individual objects.
2. Increase the variety and number of objects to which a child is exposed.

3. Improve the type of exploration or play the child exhibits with objects. For example, if the child mouths objects, work toward the child's exploration of objects with the fingers. If the child is currently banging objects, move toward the child's ability to manipulate objects in greater detail—taking off parts or putting objects in containers or holding objects appropriately (Olswang & Pinder, 1995).

TABLE 3–6. Categories of Object Play Used to Measure Developmental Progress

Categories of Play	*Behaviors that Represent Developmental Progress*
Attention Time to Object	Amount of time with an object
Type of Object Play	Mouthing
	Exploring with finger movements
	Banging
	Throwing
	Attempting to take top off/put top on
	Attempting to release object into container
	Exploring cause-effect action
	Using object functionally
Object Selection	Squeeze toys
	Textured toys
	Toys with parts
	Toys to be activated
	Functional toys

Note. Adapted from Olswang, L. B. and Pinder, G. L. (1995). Preverbal functional communication and the role of object play in children with cerebral palsy. p. 284. *Infant toddler intervention* 5(3), 277–300. Reprinted with permission of Singular Publishing Group, Inc.

TEACHING CHILDREN TO COMMUNICATE FOR A VARIETY OF REASONS

Who? Child with tracheostomy who has had limited opportunities to communicate.
What? Procedures that can be used to improve the opportunities (and the reasons) children with tracheostomies have to communicate.
When? A speech-language pathologist who is working with a child with tracheostomy in the hospital or a child who has been recently discharged from the hospital.
Where? In the home or hospital by a speech-language pathologist with help from parents.
How? Specific procedures will be outlined.
Why? Research has shown that it is important that children exhibit a variety of reasons why they communicate. Three major reasons for communicating, to regulate the behavior of others, to be social, and to establish joint attention, appear to be linked to later language development, and it is important that children exhibit reasons to communicate in each of these categories (Wetherby, Yonclas, & Bryan, 1989).

Research Support

Kertoy and Waters (1995) studied communicative intentions exhibited by three children with tracheostomies in place and who ranged in age from 20 to 27 months. All three children exhibited communicative reasons in the categories of regulation, joint attention, and social interaction, but the percentage of communicative intentions classified as regulating others' behaviors (75.5%) was four times greater than the percentage of intentions classified as social interaction (18.7%). Only a small percentage of behaviors classified as joint attention (5.6%) was exhibited by these children. The children expressed all intentions primarily through the use of gestures (gestures ranged from 68.9 to 81.3% of their total communications).

Guidelines

Speech-language pathologists can consult the goals and starting points for training a variety of communicative functions listed in Table 3–7. Several approaches can be taken:

1. The speech-language pathologist can provide and demonstrate to families a number of different situations in which the child has opportunities to use a variety of communicative functions. For example, the speech-language pathologist might model greeting the child on entering the therapy room (social function), provide the child with a choice of toy or activity for the day (behavior regulation function) and attempt to engage the child in nonverbal turn-taking with a toy to encourage the child's looking at the object and at the therapist (joint attention function).
2. The speech-language pathologist may set up specific situations in which the child needs to use various communicative functions for the activity to continue. For example, the therapist may enter the room, but wait for the child to issue the first greeting. The speech-language pathologist may bring a colorful toy box into the room, but wait for the child to request her to open the box before beginning to play.

   Or, the speech-language pathologist might engage the child in a motor activity the child likes (rocking in a rocking chair, etc.), but refuse to continue the activity until the child engages the clinician or takes a motor turn.

TABLE 3–7. Beginning Goals for Teaching Communicative Intentions in Three Major Categories

Social	*Joint Attention*	*Regulation of Others*
Goals:		
Smiles at sound or touch	Looks at objects	Protests
Smiles at self in mirror	Trys to draw attention to object	Requests actions
Smiles at familiar person	Shows object	
Issues social greetings		
Shows affection		
Starting Points:		
1. Teach Child to imitate "hi/bye" or calling out	1. Teach child to look at an object and point or make sound	Teach "yes", "no" and "want" through any communication means
2. Teach child to show affection	2. Teach child to handle an object and show it	
3. Teach child to respond in a social routine and later to initiate the routine		

Note. From Johnson-Martin, N. M., Jens, K. G., Attermeier, S. M. & Hacker, B. J. (1991). *The Carolina curriculum for infants and toddlers with special needs. Second Edition*. pp. 235–236. Reprinted with permission of Paul H. Brookes Publishing Co., Baltimore, MD.

FACILITATING SPEECH PRODUCTION FROM ORAL-MOTOR MOVEMENTS

The speech-language pathologist will want to encourage the child's use of a variety of oral movements. These movements will provide the foundation for producing a variety of vowels and consonants as well as the oral-motor skills to distinguish vowels (high vs. mid vs. low vowels). The child can be encouraged to use a variety of tongue, lip, and mouth postures to provide varied oral experiences that the child with tracheostomy may be restricted in performing. These activities can be done with or without voicing. Table 3–8 lists the oral-motor structures and control required to perform various forms of speech production (Morris, 1981). The child with tracheostomy who has been tube fed or in the hospital for an extended period may not have had opportunities to practice these oral patterns that would typically occur through feeding, oral exploration, and speech.

TABLE 3–8. Oral-Motor Movements and Control Required for Speech Production

Oral Movement and Control	*Speech Production Activity*
Inward tightening of the cheeks	Forward projection of airstream for production of fricatives
Fine motor movements of tongue-hump and/or spread	Distinctions between high, mid, and low vowels
	Production of glides and diphthongs
	Production of sibilants
Variation in lip rounding and closure	Production of round versus unround vowels, "oh" vs. "ee"
	Production of b vs. p
Forward and backward movement of the tongue	Production of distinctions between front, central, and back vowels
	Production of interdental, th
Separation of tongue and jaw movement	Rapid production of sounds requiring tongue elevation—t, d, r, j, k, g
Use of palate and posterior tongue for closure and release of back of vocal tract	Shifts from nasal to oral production
Use of lips and anterior tongue for closure and release of front of vocal tract	Production of anterior stop consonants—p, b, t, and d

Note. From Morris, S. (1981). The normal acquisition of oral feeding skills: Implications for assessment and treatment, Workshop proceedings. Boston: June 20–23, 1981.

PROCEDURE TO ENCOURAGE ORAL MOVEMENTS USED IN SPEECH PRODUCTION (WITH OR WITHOUT VOICING)

Who? The child with tracheostomy who has had limited movement of the oral structures and little opportunity for practice using the lips, jaw, or tongue.
What? Procedure to encourage oral movements used in speech production.
When? When the child has had few opportunities to vocalize or use the oral mechanism.
Where? At home or in the hospital by the speech-language pathologist.
How? A series of movement exercises to encourage oral movements that are typically needed in speech production.
Why? Because children with long-term tracheostomies may not have many opportunities to practice speech or perform the oral movements involved in speech production, the speech-language pathologist provides practice with a variety of oral movements.

Research Support

There are no studies that have investigated the provision of practice of oral movements needed in speech production of vowels and consonants on the onset or accuracy of speech production in children with tracheostomies. Children with tracheostomies require a period of time to vocalize more complex speech patterns (Bleile, 1998), and some children who have been cannulated for long periods display articulation difficulties (Kertoy, Guest, Quart, & Lieh-Lai, 1999). Because the speech production skills appear particularly vulnerable in long-term tracheostomy, the speech-language pathologist may want to encourage oral movements, even in those children who are not producing sound consistently.

Procedures

1. Model and attempt to have the child imitate some basic oral motor movements required for speech. Begin with some of the following movements:
   a. Lip rounding and lip opening ("woo" vs. "wee" or "wah")
   b. Moving tongue from back to front of mouth—tongue bunching in back, tongue spreading, tongue forward (k or g sound (back) vs. j (central) vs. s or z (front)
   c. Oral vs. nasal production (oh vs. noh)
   d. Lip smack with lower lip turned into lower lip sounds, (p, b, m, f, v or w)
2. Model separate movements and see if the child will imitate them.
3. Once the child can imitate a single movement, work on modeling more dynamic movements from front to back or high to low tongue movements.
4. If the child is reluctant to imitate the movements, try incorporating tongue and lip postures into games or songs. Pretend to be a donkey making the movements for hee-haw (wide spread lips versus open lips). Pretend to be a monkey; hump the tongue and round the lips for "hoo, hoo, hoo."

STIMULATING VOCAL PRACTICE

Who? Child with tracheostomy in place who is just beginning to vocalize.
What? Procedures that can be used to improve a child's imitation and/or spontaneous use of vocalizations.
When? A speech-language pathologist who is working with a child with tracheostomy in the hospital or at home.
Where? In the home or hospital by the speech-language pathologist with help from parents.
How? Specific procedures will be outlined.
Why? Children with tracheostomies may have limited opportunities to vocalize.

Research Support

The speech production skills of children who undergo long-term tracheostomies appear to be severely limited (Kamen & Watson, 1991; Kertoy et al., 1999). These poor speech production skills continue 6 months or longer following decannulation (Bleile, 1998). Children will use syllables and a few words for a long period of time even after decannulation (Locke & Pearson, 1990).The lack of speech practice appears to influence expressive language development because expressive skills fall far below the skills expected for the child's cognitive and receptive language abilities (Bleile, 1998, Kertoy & Morrison, 2000).

Fus and Wacker (1993) showed that one child who had undergone tracheostomy at 3 months and who wore an Airlife T adapter speaking valve benefited from a 12-week vocal stimulation program at 24 months of age. These researchers employed a single subject design that monitored the child's use of vocalizations (vowels or glottals), prespeech behaviors (lip smacking and labial sputters), and social behaviors (eye contact, smiling) during therapy sessions where the child did and did not use a speaking valve. The mean percentage of communication behaviors (all categories combined) was approximately 44% averaged for the days the child did not use the valve compared to a mean of 67% on days the child used a speaking valve. There was also an increase in social behaviors that accompanied the increase in vocalizations. The percentages were obtained from the average number of behaviors occurring in multiple, 6-second observation intervals taken from a given session.

Procedures:

When the child is able to voice sounds:

1. Start by having the child tolerate the occlusion of the stoma or a speaking valve for 5–10 minutes at a time.
2. Once the child is comfortable with occluding the stoma or wearing the speaking valve, the child is likely to connect making sounds with occlusion of the stoma and attempt to make sounds.

When the child vocalizes spontaneously:

1. Note any sounds the child makes spontaneously and also the activities or context in which sound production occurs (when sitting in high chair, when playing with a favorite toy, etc.). The potential sounds are likely to be: (a) a vowel, (b) blowing bubbles with the lips (raspberries) and/or

(c) a wide mouth vocalization made in the back of the mouth (glottal sound) and/or (d) a nasal-like hum.

2. Engage the child in interaction by establishing eye contact and smiling.

Note when the child produces any sounds spontaneously.

3. Imitate the child's vocalization.

4. Be quiet for a while and wait for the child to say the sound again.

5. If the child vocalizes, try to keep the vocal exchange going by saying what the child says again.

6. If the child does not vocalize on his/her own, model a vocalization the child is known to use.

If the child does not vocalize on his/her own, but is capable of vocalizing:

1. Try making sounds while playing with a toy. Make sounds that might be associated with the toy by children, typically:

   a. Make a glottal sound like an animal sound or growl when playing with a stuffed animal.

   b. Make a labial sputter (a raspberry like a motor engine) while pushing a car or other toy.

2. Hand the child a toy and then encourage the child to take a turn. See if the child will imitate playing with the toy or vocalizing.

3. Continue modeling sounds while playing even if the child does not vocalize. Hearing speech directed to them may encourage babbling in infants who are developing language normally (Kuhl & Meltzoff, 1982).

4. Encourage nonverbal turns at first, and then expect some sound making from the child.

5. If the child makes sounds without voice, encourage these as well. The mouthing of articulatory postures for sounds will provide some needed practice and feedback on motor movements (Meltzoff, 1986).

6. Once the child imitates sounds and/or makes sounds on his/her own, begin modeling vowels for the child (see the next section on stimulating vowel production).

The goal of these activities is to make the child comfortable with vocalizing and for the child to gain some positive regard from others for vocalizing. If vocalizing is viewed as a pleasurable and attention-getting activity, the child is likely to continue. The goal is NOT for the child to say a particular sound or sounds in the beginning.

VOCALIZING WITH A SPEAKING VALVE

The speech-language pathologist's goal of stimulating vocalizations follows an assessment of the child's ability to breathe independently and produce voicing. The issues presented in Box 3–3 outline some of the issues and decisions regarding placement of a speaking valve. For children who are not good candidates for a valve, teaching the child to occlude the stoma or produce sound with an electrolarynx will be implemented to facilitate ongoing vocal practice. (An electrolarynx may not be appropriate as an ongoing communication system, but it may help the child to make the connection between the sound source and the production of sound.)

BOX 3–3. Issues and Facts About Tracheal Tubes and Speaking Valves: Implications for Voicing and Vocalizing by Children with Tracheostomies in Place

1. The child needs to be capable of independent breathing (around the tracheal tube, or with cuff deflated) in order to produce vocalizations (Tippett, 2000).
2. The size of the tracheal tube should be approximately 2/3 the size of the tracheal lumen to allow air to escape around the tube for vocalizing (Mason & Watkins, 1992). The speech-language pathologist should have a part in the decision regarding the type of tube/ventilator that is placed in order that vocalization can be facilitated if anatomically possible. Children who require high-pressure ventilators may need a larger tracheal tube, and this will negatively affect the child's ability to vocalize (Driver, 2000).
3. The tracheal tube, ventilator and one-way speaking valve need to be compatible in size. Most tracheal tubes have a 15 mm hub on which the speaking valve will fit. If the tube is not standard size, adapters can be ordered to fit the speaking valve to the tracheal tube.
4. Children who are ventilated as well as tracheostomized can use speaking valves. There are several speaking valves that are specifically made to go with ventilators: Passy-Muir Speaking Valve (Passy-Muir, Inc.), Montgomery Tracheostomy Speaking Valve (Boston Medical Products), and the Hood Speaking Valve (Hood Laboratories).
5. Placement of a one-way speaking valve is generally a team decision made by the speech-language pathologist, respiratory therapist, family, and physician. Written medical documentation is needed prior to ordering and placing the valve.
6. The amount of secretions produced by the child will likely be reduced with the speaking valve. Some children with excessive secretions may be hindered in the use of a valve. The speech-language pathologist must know and follow the hospital or home care procedures specified for suctioning a particular child.
7. Cuffed tracheal tubes are not usually recommended for children because they may damage tracheal tissue and may not be needed, since children have tracheas that are small in diameter. If a cuffed tracheal tube is necessary, generally foam or silicone cuffs are used. Foam cuffs may not be appropriate for use with speaking valves because they tend to inflate/deflate automatically with the breathing cycle (Driver, 2000).
8. The speech-language pathologist will need to know the pressure levels recommended for each patient. When the child wears a valve, the airflow patterns change, and adjustments will likely be needed in the pressure levels. It is advised that the speech-language pathologist work in conjunction with the respiratory therapist and physician when the valve is initially placed in order that appropriate pressure levels can be established (See Resource Section—Respiration).
9. Children will likely experience some discomfort in the beginning. The child's comfort level may be influenced by trapping of air and improper settings on the ventilator for number of breaths per minute or volume levels (Mason & Watkins, 1992). The speech-language pathologist should work together with the respiratory therapist to establish the appropriate settings for each child (See glossary for definitions of some key terms).

STIMULATING VOWEL PRODUCTION

Who? Child with tracheostomy in place who is vocalizing.
What? Procedures that can be used to improve a child's imitation and spontaneous use of vowels.
When? When a speech-language pathologist wants to increase the amount of vocalizing or the clarity or strength of vowel production.
Where? In the home or hospital by the speech-language pathologist with help from the parents.
How? Specific procedures will be outlined. The goal is to move the child through the developmental sequence of sound production.
Why? Some children with tracheostomies have been shown to exhibit poor speech sound production, including poor production of vowels (Kamen & Watson, 1991).

Research Support

Kamen and Watson (1991) showed that a group of children with long-term tracheostomies had difficulties with production of the vowel [i] (F1 and F2 formant frequencies) and with production of [a] (F1 formant frequency) compared to their peers who had not undergone tracheostomies. These children with tracheostomies had a tendency to neutralize vowels, substituting the central vowel [^] for others. Although vowel production difficulties have been shown to occur in children with tracheostomies, there have been no intervention studies to document the efficacy of stimulating the use of vowels in children with tracheostomies.

Procedures:

1. Note any vowels that a child vocalizes.
2. Note if the child produces vowels to mark each of the vowel quadrants and follows the developmental sequence of vowel production (see Developmental Sequence in Table 3–9).
3. Model vowels that the child currently uses.
4. Wait for the child to imitate the sounds.
5. Note if the child will imitate these vowels.
6. Use vowels that the child is comfortable producing and work on varying the length or volume at which the vowels are produced. Can the child hold production of the vowel for a longer period of time? Can the child increase the loudness with which the vowel is produced?

   First, try to increase the usage of vowels that the child is currently using and have the child become comfortable taking vocal turns with you. Play games to see who can say the longest or loudest or lowest or highest-pitched vowel. By having the child vary loudness, length, and pitch, he or she gains greater motor control over vocal and oral functioning.

   Next, introduce new vowels for the child to produce.

7. The speech-language pathologist may want to introduce/model for the child to imitate:

a. Vowels in the order of occurrence in the developmental sequence (Refer to Table 3–9).

b. Other vowels that exhibit similar parameters to vowels the child can produce.

For example, if a child produces the mid, unrounded, tense, front vowel [e], but not the high, unrounded, tense, front vowel [i], try stimulating production of [i].

c. Lax vowels [ɛ], [I], [æ], [o] or [ʊ]. Lax vowels were used most frequently by children from 3–14 months (Lieberman, 1980).

d. The vowel [u] before [i] or [a] if none of these is currently used. The vowels [i] and [a] are more difficult for children with tracheostomy to produce than [u] (Kamen and Watson, 1991).

8. Provide models of vowels *only* at first. Vowel production may be influenced by the consonants that follow. If vowels are modeled in VC or CVC contexts, vary the consonants that are paired with the vowels (Pollack, 1991).

TABLE 3–9. Developmental Sequence of Vowel Acquisition

Timing of Acquisition	*Vowels Acquired*
Early	i, a, u, o, ʌ
Mid	æ,ʊ,ɔ,ə
Late	e,ɛ,I,ɚ,ɝ

Note. From Stoel-Gammon, C. and Herrington, P. (1990). Vowel systems of normally developing and phonologically disordered children. *Clinical Linguistics and Phonetics, 4*, 145–160. Reprinted with permission of Taylor and Francis, Ltd., London, UK.

USING PAIRS OF VOWELS TO IMPROVE VOWEL PRODUCTION

The studies of vowel production in children with tracheostomies in place suggest that these children produce many vowels, but that their vowels are imprecise (Kamen & Watson, 1991; Kertoy et al., 1999). Therefore, a procedure such as the following prescribed by Bauman-Waengler (2000) appears appropriate for helping children with tracheostomies recognize distinctions between the vowels they produce and the correct production. The tracheal tube is thought to restrict tongue placement, which can result in poor tongue placement in the front of the mouth and/or a lack of tongue elevation (Kamen & Watson, 1991).

Procedures to Stimulate Vowels and Vowel Pairs:

Procedures are based on techniques outlined by Bauman-Waengler (2000).

1. Count the child's vowel errors and note the vowel(s) that are produced incorrectly most frequently.
2. Note the vowels that are substituted for the target vowel.
3. Pair a substitute vowel the child produces with the target vowel.

   For example, if the child substitutes the mid central vowel, [ʌ] for the high front vowel, [i]. Word pairs might include:

   hut - heat　　tum - teem

   mut - meet　　bum - beam

   sum - seem

   Children who are developing language normally would be expected to show increasing variation in their use of vowels from 4–6 months of age (Proctor, 1989).

MOTOR MOVEMENTS FOR VOWEL PRODUCTION

Speech-language pathologists may also want to attend to the motor movements associated with vowel production that create distinct differences between vowels. Because children with tracheostomies may experience confusion with tongue placement for vowels because of long periods with a tracheal tube in place, speech-language pathologists should consider the tongue and lip movements needed for correct vowel production (see Box 3–4). Some children with tracheostomies may have imprecise vowels due to the extended period in which the tongue was carried in a retracted position in the vocal tract (Kamen and Watson, 1991)

BOX 3–4. Tongue and Lip Placement for Vowel Production

Front versus back vowels—part of the tongue that is elevated
High versus low vowels—how high the tongue is elevated toward the palate
Rounded versus unrounded—the rounding of the lips

PROVIDING INTERVENTION ONCE THE TRACHEOSTOMY IS REMOVED

Because the recovery of speech and language in children following decannulation can proceed slowly over months or even years, children and their families will continue to require the services of speech-language pathologists. Speech-language pathologists can conduct direct services and/or consult with families about integrating speech and language activities into everyday routines. The speech-language pathologist will want to focus on the following speech and language goals, based on research findings about speech and language characteristics of children who experience long-term tracheostomies:

1. Increasing the rate and complexity of a child's vocalizations.
2. Improving the phonological abilities of children.
3. Stimulating expressive language skills.

INCREASING THE RATE OF VOCALIZATIONS FOLLOWING TRACHEOSTOMY

Who? The child who is decannulated, but who is not vocalizing on a frequent basis.
What? Procedures that can be used to increase a child's rate of vocalizing.
When? A speech-language pathologist who is working with a child following tracheostomy and who has concerns that the child is not vocalizing at a frequent rate.
Where? In the home by the speech-language pathologist with help from parents.
How? Specific procedures will be outlined.
Why? Children have shown slower than normal rates of vocalizing while tracheostomized and following decannulation (Locke & Pearson, 1990). The rate of vocalizing prior to 1 year of age has been strongly correlated with later advancements in language and cognitive development (Stoel-Gammon, 1992).

Research Support

Four children, who were tracheostomized, vocalized far less frequently than children who are developing language normally (Morrison, 1998). These subjects ranged in mean vocalizations per minute from 1.15 (Subject 1 at 20–21 months corrected age) to 4.82 vocalizations per minute (Subject 4 at 20–21 months corrected age). Camp, Burgess, Morgan, and Zerbe (1987) showed that children who were developing language normally vocalized at a mean rate of 3.86 vocalization per minute at 2 months to a mean rate of 7.92 vocalizations per minute at 12 months.

Procedures

For the child who is tracheostomized, the goal is to elicit vocalizations, but for the child who is no longer tracheostomized, the goal is to increase the number of vocalizations. The speech-language pathologist will want to work with the family to determine times and situations in which the child is most likely to vocalize. The family should be encouraged to interact with the child and to stimulate vocalizing. Any of the following situations might serve as appropriate situations for stimulating vocalizations within interactions. The child may use mainly CV syllables and a few words for a long while after decannulation (Bleile, 1998). It is important to increase the amount of vocalizing at the child's current level, while encouraging vocalizations at the next level of complexity.

Expect the Child to Vocalize

Encourage families to expect vocalizations from the child with tracheostomy as they would from other children in appropriate situations.

Imitation

When the child vocalizes, imitate what he/she has said. Wait and expect the child to vocalize again. Try to engage the child in vocal turn-taking.

Routines

Children may vocalize more frequently during bathtime or other daily routines. Begin to pair the vocalizations the child uses in specific situations with those familiar activities. Imitate and reinforce these vocalizations.

Songs or Rhymes or Books

Sing songs or read books that have sounds in them that young children could easily say and join the adult in unison. The adult could read from the book, *Brown Bear, Brown Bear, What Do You See?* (Martin & Carle, 1995). The adult could have the child join in to produce the [b] in bear or the [m] in the response, I see an alligator looking at me! Or the parent could read from Dr. Seuss's book, *Green Eggs and Ham* (Seuss, 1960) and emphasize production of "I" or "you" in the following phrases. "I do not like green eggs and ham, I'm Sam I am" ("I" occurs several times). "Would you, could eat it ....?" ("you" occurs several times). Books provide multiple exemplars of the sounds and multiple opportunities to expect a response from the child. A list of books that stimulate various language structures is outlined in Paul, 1995 (see resources for complete reference).

INCREASING THE NUMBER OF CONSONANTS PRODUCED FOLLOWING TRACHEOSTOMY

Who? The child who is decannulated, but who is producing mostly vowels and some consonant + vowel combinations.
What? Procedures that can be used to improve the number of consonants produced by children after decannulation.
When? A speech-language pathologist who is working with a child following tracheostomy and who has concerns that the child is not producing a variety of consonants appropriate for his/her age.
Where? In the home by the speech-language pathologist with help from parents.
How? Specific procedures will be outlined.
Why? Children who have been tracheostomized for a long period of time begin to vocalize when the tracheal tube is removed, but progress in producing a variety of consonants is slow.

Research Support

Locke and Pearson (1990) showed that at 6 weeks following decannulation, a subject of 20 months used five different consonants. Bleile (1998) found that a 32-month old subject used four different consonants 4 months after decannulation, similar to the number of consonants produced by children at 15 months of age. These two children showed a preference for use of labial consonants. These studies show that the speech production skills of children remain severely restricted and are well below age expectations for a period of time following decannulation. There have been no studies investigating improvements in consonant production brought about by vocal or consonant stimulation in children with tracheostomies.

Procedures

1. Prepare a transcription of the vocalizations or words used by the child.
2. Note the number of different consonants used and the sound classes that are represented.
3. Select other consonants from sound classes similar to those represented in the inventory for training. For example, if the child uses one or two stops, select other stops for training.
4. Provide models of those consonants to the child and note if the child will imitate them. Next, introduce objects and events that contain sounds the child would be expected to use. Following this, provide opportunities for the child to learn the names of the objects or events.
5. Next, select books or songs or a favorite toy that contains sounds the child is likely to use. Suggest to the family that they read the books to the child or interact with the child with the toy so that the child has numerous opportunities to hear the sound(s).

INCREASING THE COMPLEXITY OF SYLLABLES FOLLOWING TRACHEOSTOMY

Who? The child who is decannulated and who is producing consonants.
What? Procedures that can be used to improve the complexity of the vocalizations produced by children after decannulation.
When? When a speech-language pathologist who is working with a child following tracheostomy has concerns that the child is not producing complex syllables or words.
Where? In the home by the speech-language pathologist with help from parents.
How? Specific procedures will be outlined.
Why? Children who have been tracheostomized for a long period of time begin to vocalize when the tracheal tube is removed, but make slow progress toward producing complex productions.

Research Support

Support for the child's use of a variety of consonants at an early age comes from a number of sources. Stoel-Gammon (1992) showed that children who have a large number of consonants in their inventories at an early age have significantly larger vocabularies at an earlier age than children who take longer to establish an inventory with diverse consonants. This is presumably because children who can produce a greater number of consonants have more consonants from which to make potential words. Vihman and Greenlee (1987) studied children at ages 1 and 3 years and showed that those children who were more accurate in their early consonant production, also had fewer errors in production 2 years later. Vihman (1992) studied several groups of infants (English, as well as French, Swedish, and Japanese), who varied in age from 9 to 24 months of age, through the period of development of 50 words. She showed that the syllable shapes the children used were dependent on (a) the salience of the models in the adult language and (b) how motorically accessible the syllables were for the children. Some children preferred to use a number of diverse syllable types with different consonants, while others used the same pattern repeatedly. The children who were not as advanced tended to use syllables with easier motor movements, that is, producing a back vowel and consonant together to reduce tongue movement.

These research findings suggest that the use of consonants and complex syllables serve a role in later word production. Children may take different routes in moving from syllable to word production. The amount of progress made by children with tracheostomies may be dependent in part on their readiness to motorically produce diverse syllable types. With stimulation, speech-language pathologists can encourage those children who are ready.

Procedures

1. Teach consonants (likely labials) that the child is currently using in syllables of increasing complexity.
2. Note vowels that are facilitated by the surrounding consonants—back vowels with velars or high front vowels with alveolars (Davis and MacNeilage, 1990).
3. Begin with open CVs.
4. Continue with repetition of the same CV to produce more complex syllables, CVCV, as these syllables may be less motorically complex for the child to produce.
5. Continue with closed syllables with two consonants.
6. Take care in selecting the multiple consonants to be used in single and multiple syllables. Issues to consider include:
   a. Use consonants the child is comfortable producing. Young children have been found to use syllables and words that contain sounds they can produce and to avoid words with sounds that are not yet in their repertoire.
   b. Are both consonants voiced or unvoiced? Some children with tracheostomies show confusions with the plus/minus voice distinction (Kertoy, et al., 1999). Use of consonants with similar voicing features may be helpful, for example, bad, dab rather than bat or dat or baba or dada rather than tada or taka.
   c. Be aware of the movement transition the child is required to make. If children with tracheostomies are experiencing difficulties with the timing of movements or with accurate tongue placement, then selecting syllables with consonants that require easy movement transitions might facilitate easier production. Velleman and Strand (1998) have applied this principle for use with children with apraxia. For example, have the child produce syllables in which he/she moves from a labial to a labial or from a labial to an alveolar rather than from a bilabial to a velar (requiring a movement from front to back). Examples of syllables with bilabial to bilabial transitions might include: m-b, b-m, p-m, m-m, etc. Examples of syllables with bilabial to alveolar transitions might include: p-t, b-d, b-t, b-n, w-d, etc.

SYLLABLE AND CONSONANT COMPLEXITY CHART

The grid employed by Velleman and Strand (1998), displayed in Table 3–10, may be useful to the speech-language pathologist for stimulating increasingly more complex syllables in children with tracheostomies.

TABLE 3–10. Syllable and Consonant Complexity Chart

		Number of consonants			
		1	2	3	4
Number of syllables	1	open CV (ma)a	closed CVC (pam)		
	2		open CVCV (mama)	closed CVCVC (pie pan)	
	3			open CVCVCV (paperboy)	closed CVCVCVC (baby bed)

Note. From Velleman, S. L. and Strand, K. E. (1998). *Dynamic remediation strategies for children with developmental verbal dyspraxia*. American Speech-Language-Hearing Association. Reprinted with permission of the American Speech-Language-Hearing Association, Rockville, MD.

a = Examples provided in parentheses

IMPROVING THE PHONOLOGICAL ABILITIES OF CHILDREN FOLLOWING TRACHEOSTOMIES

Who? The child who is decannulated, is vocalizing, but who exhibits multiple sound errors.
What? Procedures that can be used to improve the phonological abilities of children after decannulation.
When? When a speech-language pathologist is working with a child following tracheostomy and has concerns about the child's sound production skills.
Where? In the home by the speech-language pathologist with help from parents.
How? Specific procedures will be outlined.
Why? Children who have been tracheostomized for a long period of time, begin to vocalize when the tracheal tube is removed, but make slow progress toward complex productions. These children may show residual phonological difficulties (Kertoy, et al., 1999; Ross, 1982; Simon, Fowler, & Handler, 1983).

Research Support

Kertoy et al. (1999) showed that six children with long-term tracheotomies exhibited several phonological processes in greater than 40% of opportunities, as measured by the *Assessment of Phonological Processes-Revised* (Hodson, 1986). The most prominent process was stridency deletion, used by 5 of 6 children, followed by liquid deviation (used in greater than 70% of opportunities) by 4 of 6 children and cluster reduction used by 3 of 6 children. Two children exhibited postvocalic obstruent omission and velar deviation in greater than 40% of opportunities. All six children, four who ranged in age from 2;8 to 3;3 years, and two who were aged 6;4 and 6;8 years, exhibited stridency deletion and liquid deviation. The four younger children exhibited cluster reduction, velar deviation and postvocalic obstruent omission. Two of the children remained cannulated at the time of the study and two children had been decannulated within 3 months of the study. This may have contributed to the prevalent use of processes.

Hill and Singer (1990) documented widespread articulation difficulties in 61% of children with tracheostomies between the ages of 2;1 and 8;6 years. Some of the children studied (29%) were born prematurely, and some also exhibited CNS complications (43%). The types of articulation errors were not specified in their study. Ross (1982) documented the occurrence of some articulation/phonology errors in three children with normal cognitive skills who underwent long-term tracheostomies. All three children showed difficulties with consonant blends, one with final consonant deletion, and one with an [f] for [p] substitution.

Simon, Fowler, and Handler (1983) documented phonological difficulties in 15 children who had been tracheostomized long term, and the phonological difficulties required treatment. Eleven of 15 children showed significant improvement in sound production with treatment. This study is the only study to document the efficacy of treating phonological skills in children with tracheostomies. The study did not employ a control group of children with tracheostomies who did not receive treatment to note if some children would have improved without treatment.

Making Clinical Decisions

There are several clinical implications of the studies that have investigated the phonological characteristics of children with tracheostomies. The types of processes shown by multiple subjects, stridency deletion and liquid deviation, involve sound classes and distinctions that are acquired later. These patterns may suggest that these children with tracheostomies are simply slow to develop the sound system of their language and that these skills will be acquired gradually. The speech-language pathologist may employ a phonological process approach to stimulate numerous sounds and to bring out broad changes in the child's system in a short period of time. The age of the child and the number of processes exhibited in greater than 40% of opportunities should be important factors when deciding to treat. The older child who exhibits multiple processes should be treated.

In some children, a phonetic approach to treatment may be appropriate (Secord, 1985). It is not known if articulatory factors contribute to the phonological patterns shown by some children with tracheostomies. For example, do children have difficulty with stridents because of the feature of continuant? Do children with tracheostomies have difficulty maintaining sounds of ongoing duration? Or do some children have difficulty with liquids and some stridents because of the dynamic tongue positions required to produce these sounds? These issues should be considered by clinician as potential factors to be ruled out when treating children with tracheostomies.

Children who show difficulty with tongue placement for particular sounds might benefit from a phonetic approach. The speech-language pathologist should judge the best treatment for a child based on the child's errors and recognize that no studies have been conducted to support the efficacy of any one approach.

Procedures For the Child with Multiple Sound Errors

1. Administer the *Assessment of Phonological Processes-Revised* (Hodson, 1986) pre- and posttreatment.

2. Note processes that occur with greater than 40% accuracy. Select processes for treatment that should have been repressed by the child's age, that occur with frequency, and/or that contribute to poor intelligibility.
3. Follow particular guidelines for treatment of phonological processes outlined by Hodson and Paden (1991).
4. Clinicians may also want to pursue a distinctive feature approach if stridents are involved (Blache, 1989). Children with tracheostomies may benefit from training that distinguishes between +strident (f, s) and –strident (th) features.
5. If children exhibit sounds that are resistant to treatment, then the clinician might review if there are any patterns to the sound errors and if they are influenced by place of articulation. Phonetic placement techniques may be beneficial for some children.

IMPROVING EXPRESSIVE LANGUAGE ABILITIES FOLLOWING TRACHEOSTOMIES

Who? The child who is decannulated, but who exhibits delays in expressive language skills.
What? Decision-making and content areas for improving expressive language abilities of children after decannulation.
When? When a speech-language pathologist who is working with a child following tracheostomy and has concerns about a child's expressive language functioning (assessment shows a discrepancy between receptive and expressive language skills).
Where? In the home by the speech-language pathologist with help from parents.
How? Specific issues to enhance decision-making and content areas for improving expressive language will be outlined.
Why? Many children who have been tracheostomized for a long period of time exhibit expressive language delays (Ross, 1982).

Research Support

Simon, Fowler, and Handler (1983) documented the expressive language skills of nine children who were tracheostomized from the prelinguistic period into the linguistic period. These children were cannulated from 10 to 31 months and had little or no opportunity to vocalize. Only two of the nine children had expressive language skills within the normal range, while seven children showed expressive language delays. Three subjects exhibited severe delays of greater than several years, and four children showed delays of 4 to 10 months in expressive language skills.

Ross (1982) assessed six children for expressive language skills. Three of the children showed below average cognitive skills in addition to expressive language delays. The three children with cognitive functioning within the normal range, showed mixed language functioning. Two of the three exhibited near normal expressive language skills, with numerous errors in morphology and syntax. One of the three exhibited language skills below age level expectations, with deficiencies in sentence length and complexity.

Making Clinical Decisions

The clinician has little information on which to base intervention goals for children with expressive language delays according to language characteristics cited in the literature for children who are tracheostomized. We know that the child with tracheostomy is at risk for severe expressive language difficulties, but to date, the nature of the expressive delays have not been well documented. Some children may need treatment in basic areas such as vocabulary development and the formulation of grammatical sentences. It is suspected that most children will show some difficulties with morphological and syntactic skills given the protracted developmental period in which these various skills are acquired. Therefore, the following guidelines are based on the little information that we currently have about those morphological and syntactic structures shown to be affected in children with tracheostomies and expressive language delays.

Procedures

Content

1. Determine the child's mean length of utterance.
2. Note the morphological and grammatical structures that correspond with the mean length of utterance.
3. Determine the child's strengths and weaknesses for his/her language level.
4. Select several goals from the child's weaker areas.
5. Based on descriptions of expressive language provided in the literature, the following morphological and syntactic areas may require treatment (Ross, 1982):
   a. Use of articles
   b. Use of auxiliary verbs
   c. Proper use of verb tense
   d. Proper subject-verb agreement
   e. Formation of grammatical sentences with subject, verb, object, and ordering.
   f. Formation of irregular third person plural.
   g. Formation of irregular past tense.

Process

1. Teach morphological and syntactic skills within natural, interactive situations.
2. Adults should provide multiple models of the target.
3. Expect responses of the target from the child within the interactions.
4. See Owens (1999) for specific procedures for teaching various morphological and syntactic structures.

SECTION 4

CASE STUDIES

TOPIC 1: VARIABILITY IN DEVELOPMENTAL PERFORMANCE OF CHILDREN WITH TRACHEOSTOMIES

The following cases exemplify typical precipitating reasons for tracheostomy along with the broad spectrum of speech and language and other developmental skills that may be exhibited by children with tracheostomies. This variability needs to be recognized by speech-language pathologists when working with children with tracheostomies as well as when helping families to set realistic expectations for their children. The complexity and content of treatment plans may vary considerably from one child to the next, but all children share the common treatment goals: the need for early intervention and the need for opportunities to communicate and vocalize.

Child 1, Background

Tim was born prematurely at 34 weeks gestation, weighing 3 pounds, 6 ounces, with bronchopulmonary dysplasia. He spent the first 9 months of life in the hospital. Tim's respiratory difficulties required a high-pressure ventilator that limited the leakage of air around his tracheostomy and his opportunities to vocalize. Tim suffered from a mild, Grade 1, intracranial bleed within the first few months in hospital, and his cognitive functioning may have been affected (Nelson, 1993).

Child 1, Risks to Speech and Language

Tim's early development places him at risk for speech and language delay for several reasons: (a) his prematurity and low birth weight; (b) his hypoxia which may affect cognition and, in turn, language development, although many children with Grade 1 bleeds have subsequent normal development (Bennett, Silver, Leung, & Mack, 1990); (c) his long-term hospitalization; and (d) his inability to vocalize at all or to receive feedback from his own vocal productions. Children at this birth weight can experience good developmental outcomes (Goldson, 1996). Tim's outcome for speech and language is dependent on development of a communication system; a sign system should be instituted if opportunities to vocalize will not be realized in the near future.

Child 2, Background

Penny was born full term with an airway obstruction subglottally that necessitated a tracheostomy to improve airflow and to maintain a patent airway. She is now 8 months of age and in stable health. The doctors will complete a laryngotracheotomy to increase the diameter of the trachea and larynx. The surgeons anticipate that Penny can then be weaned from the tracheostomy.

Child 2, Risks to Speech and Language

Penny's limited opportunities to vocalize place her at risk for speech and language delays. However, she is alert and responsive to family and staff; communicating intentionally with gestures and single signs. Her cognitive skills appear near age level, based on informal testing of symbolic play skills. If the inability to vocalize can be overcome within the next few months, Penny has a good chance for positive speech and language outcomes.

Child 3, Background

Jessie was born at 25 weeks gestation, weighing approximately 1 pound, 6 ounces. She was hospitalized for the first 10 months of her life. She required a gastronomy tube for feeding and NICU care for very-low-birth-weight infants. She underwent a tracheostomy at 3.5 months to improve clearing of secretions from the lungs and airway and for long-term ventilation. Jessie was diagnosed with spastic quadriplegia cerebral palsy at 18 months. Speech and physical therapy as well as nursing services were delivered in the home after discharge from the hospital. A speaking valve was placed at 20 months. Oral feedings have been successful and some vowels and squealing (to signal others) are occurring.

Child 3, Risks to Speech and Language

Jessie is at significant risk for speech and language delay as well as delays in other developmental areas due to her very low birth weight. She will require long-term follow-up and intervention by a speech-language pathologist. Nearly half of infants born with very low birth weight will experience some significant developmental delays (Goldson, 1996). Outcomes in the speech and language area will be influenced by: (a) her cognitive level, yet to be determined (careful, sequential evaluation is required to ensure valid outcomes with Jessie's potential motor limitations that affect her ability to complete some test items), (b) Jessie's motor functioning as it relates to respiration to support clear, sustained speech, and (c) general developmental progression in all areas of social, motor, adaptive functioning as these relate to speech and language development. Intensive, ongoing services will be required to meet Jessie's needs for an appropriate communication system as her development progresses and for her transition to school. Interdisciplinary programming with the family as a team member is essential.

Child 4, Background

Paul was diagnosed with Pierre Robin Syndrome shortly after birth. He was born full term with a small mandible and cleft of the palate. Paul experienced early problems with feeding and aspiration of food, and an airway obstruction was found. A tracheostomy was placed at 28 days of life to create a patent airway. Feeding by gastrostomy tube was needed initially, but oral feedings were gradually established. Paul was followed by an interdisciplinary feeding team at the hospital to help wean him from the gastrostomy tube to oral feeds. He is now gaining weight and is responsive to his family. He initiates communication with gestures. Informal testing of his receptive language shows near age level functioning at 12 months. The small size of the trachea and obstruction resulted in a tight fitting tracheal tube which makes vocalizing on air leakage unlikely until Paul grows.

Child 4, Risks to Speech and Language

That Paul was born full term and that he is exhibiting age appropriate receptive language skills are positive indicators for speech and language development. The combined factors of tracheostomy and cleft palate may negatively affect speech and language development.

Paul appears to be a potential candidate for a signing system, based on his spontaneous use of gestures. Speech-language pathologists will follow Paul closely and work with his family because surgeries for repair of the cleft and airway obstructions will be necessary (Lehman, Fishman, & Neiman, 1995). Use of an electrolarynx may allow for some opportunities to vocalize until structural limitations are overcome. Paul's case also illustrates the need for monitoring of the potential for airway obstruction in children with Pierre Robin Syndrome and its impact on feeding (Prodoehl & Shuttuck, 1995). The speech-language pathologist will be involved with feeding as well as speech programming in these cases.

TOPIC 2: SPEECH AND LANGUAGE ASSESSMENT WITH A TRACHEOSTOMY IN PLACE: INTERPRETING TEST RESULTS AND MAKING ONGOING ASSESSMENT DECISIONS

Case Background

Sarah was 32 months old when a speech and language assessment was conducted. She was born prematurely and intubated at birth to support her breathing. Sarah has bronchopulmonary dysplasia that required hospitalization for the first 3 months of life and several repeat hospitalizations. Sarah has tracheomalacia, which required tracheotomy at 6 months of age to create a patent airway. Sarah remains cannulated and vocalizes some by occluding her stoma. She has not received speech or language intervention.

Speech and Language Assessment

Sarah was administered the *Preschool Language Scale-3 (PLS-3:* Zimmerman, Steiner, & Pond, 1992) and the *Assessment of Phonological Processes—Revised* (*APP-R:* Hodson, 1986). A phonetic inventory was also completed from single-word utterances from a speech sample elicited during structured storybook and scripted play activities.

Assessment Results

Sarah received an age equivalent of 2 years on the Auditory Comprehension portion of the *PLS-3* and an age equivalent of 1 year, 6 months on the Expressive Communication section of the test. Her standard scores of 80 (confidence interval 74–86) and 69 (confidence interval 64–74) on the Receptive and Expressive sections of the test, respectively, place her at –1 to –1.5 standard deviations below age level expectations for receptive language and at –2 standard deviations below age expectations for expressive language.

Sarah uses primarily single words and some common two-word phrases to communicate. She understands the names of objects and common actions. She is beginning to understand what to do with objects and part/whole relationships with objects. She does not exhibit understanding of pronouns except for "me" nor understanding of quantities of objects. She understands the concept, big, but not other concepts associated with objects and people; that is, wet, dirty, round, etc.

Her phonetic inventory lacked the following sounds: [s], [z], [ʃ], [tʃ], [ʒ], [ð], [r], and [ɚ]. Sarah used approximately 68% of the 25 English consonants. Sarah exhibited the following phonological process with these percentages of occurrence on the *APP-R:*

Process	Percentage of Occurrence
Postvocalic Obstruent Omission	55%
Stridency Deletion	75%
Liquid Deviation (R)	90%
Glide Deviation	45%
Cluster Reduction	55%

Sarah received a phonological deviancy score of 32, corresponding to a Moderate severity rating on the *APP-R.* Those processes that are used in greater than 40% of opportunities and liquid deviation in greater than 70% of opportunities are generally targeted for treatment (Hodson & Paden, 1991).

Analysis of Results/Rationale for Interpretations

Those children who score greater than –1 standard deviation below the mean on standardized tests of language development are of concern to speech-language pathologists and are frequent candidates for language treatment. Sarah's performance in both receptive and expressive language are well below age expectations. Restrictions on Sarah's ability to talk places her at a severe disadvantage on tests like the *PLS-3*, where passing language items at a given age is dependent on the client's ability to give verbal responses (naming pictures, talking in sentences, etc.). That Sarah also shows receptive language skills commensurate with a child of 2 years of age is a concern.

Sarah also shows excessive use of phonological processes, with four processes used in greater than 40% of opportunities. Her phonological deviancy score indicated a moderate phonological problem. The processes of stridency deletion and liquid deviation are not repressed until an older age in children, but processes such as postvocalic obstruent omission are frequently repressed by 3 years of age. The percentages of occurrence of processes exhibited by Sarah were greater than those of children who are developing normally at 2.2 to 2.5 years studied by Preisser, Hodson, and Paden (1988).

What Should Be Done Next?

Because of the potential impact of cognitive or hearing difficulties on language development, testing should be conducted in these areas to rule out cognitive delay or hearing loss. Sarah should be referred to an audiologist for hearing testing if this has not been completed previously. Cognition may be assessed through use of the *Kaufman Brief Assessment Battery for Children* (Kaufman & Kaufman, 1983), which is appropriate for use with children 30 months to 12 years. Nonverbal cognition and symbolic play skills may be assessed through use of the *Symbolic Play Test* (Lowe & Costello, 1988), which is appropriate for use with children 12 to 36 months of age.

More extensive assessment of receptive vocabulary, object knowledge and comprehension of sentence meaning should be conducted to determine strengths and weaknesses in receptive language. The *MacArthur Communicative Development Inventories* (Fenson et al., 1996) as well as an informal test of functional use of objects (Bates, et al., 1989), which is outlined in Section 2, "Assessment," are appropriate starting points.

Consultation with the physician and family regarding the child's potential for vocalization and proposed length of cannulation would be useful for the speech-language pathologist in facilitating expressive language development. If Sarah is to remain cannulated for any additional length of time, the possibility of her wearing a speaking valve or other communication options should be pursued.

Treatment Plan Based on Assessment Results

Sarah is a candidate for treatment in receptive language and speech production. Following the outcome of additional testing, treatment options should be discussed with the family and a program established for Sarah. An ideal program would involve the parents and other professionals who visit Sarah at home and would include demonstrations of activities and goals by the speech-language pathologist and discussion of realistic ways for the family to stimulate Sarah's language comprehension and opportunities to vocalize within daily routines.

TOPIC 3: ONE CHILD'S STORY: PERSPECTIVES OF A PARENT AND A SPEECH-LANGUAGE PATHOLOGIST REGARDING CARE OVER A FIVE-YEAR PERIOD

THE CASE OF DANNY

The following were observations made by Danny's mother:

Three Days of Age, Danny in NICU

Danny is so tiny, but he is alive. He is in that room with all those wires and beeping machines. It is all so frightening. I am supposed to go home from the hospital tomorrow, but I can't leave him. I feel so guilty. Danny's dad says it isn't my fault, but I still feel like there must be something I could have done to prevent this.

Danny at 1 Month

Danny is 1 month old today. I wasn't sure he would make it this long. They had to operate and put a tube down his throat, because he couldn't breathe. Danny's doctor says he will have a much easier time trying to breathe now.

Danny at 4 Months

Danny is doing much better and is gaining weight. He is starting to respond to us now when we come. I'm sure that he recognizes us. The speech therapist is helping us to learn Danny's way of communicating with us. We are starting to see who Danny is.

Danny at 7 Months

Danny was able to take some food through his mouth today. He didn't spit it out. The speech therapist is encouraging Danny to talk by placing a buzzing machine, an electrolarynx, against his throat. The physical therapist also does some exercises with Danny to help him to sit up and support himself.

Danny at 10 Months

We are so excited because Danny came home 2 days ago. We are also exhausted, because we have been afraid to sleep for fear we wouldn't hear him if he needed help. Today the nurse brought a monitor that we can keep in our bedroom to alert us if Danny wakes up in the night.

Danny at 18 Months

I feel guilty, but sometimes I just want to close the door and ask all the people who come to the house for Danny to go home. I am thankful for their help and Danny is making progress, but it is so hard to give up our privacy. Sometimes they forget that this is our home. I guess that's the way it will have to be for a while longer.

Danny at 2 Years

Danny will celebrate his second birthday next week. We have come a long way. Danny is making some sounds and learning to sign. He is walking a little and pulling his ventilator along behind him. His grandma comes every Tuesday when the physical therapist visits, and grandma helps him with his motor program. We couldn't have made it if Nan and Pappap didn't live just down the street and help us out with Danny and his older brother.

Danny at 2½ Years

I am taking a signing course so I can use more signs with Danny. His speech is still weak and breathy.

Danny at 3 Years

Danny got a speaking valve that fits on his ventilator 4 weeks ago. He is starting to adjust to it and is able to make a few, very clear sounds. His speech seems stronger. We allowed Danny to be part of a research project to look at his speech with his speaking valve. Danny's father and I wanted to give something back for all the help and support we have received from the professional staff who visit us at home.

Danny at 5 Years

Danny will start school at a special preschool where he will receive speech, occupational, and physical therapy daily and interact with other children. Some of them have special needs. I went to talk to the teacher last week and she had lots of questions about Danny's ventilator. I told Danny's teacher that if I could learn what to do that she could as well. The speech and respiratory therapists have set up a training program for the teacher so she can monitor Danny's ventilator in class. I'm glad that Danny will be able to get all his therapies at school. I couldn't imagine transporting him to each therapist!

The following observations were taken from the case notes made by Danny's speech-language pathologist:

Danny at 1 Month

I visited Danny and his family in the NICU today. I introduced myself and let the family know I was available to answer any questions they might have when they were ready. I told them I would be working with the respiratory therapist, who is serving as Danny's case manager and coordinator of Danny's treatment team.

Danny at 4 Months

I visited Danny and his mother in the NICU today. His mother and I used the "Observation of Signals Checklist," and Mrs. Brown quickly picked up on Danny's signals. Mrs. Brown also observed how I demonstrated a response to Danny when he looked at her and smiled.

Danny at 11 Months

I visited Danny and Mrs. Brown in the Browns' home today. Mrs. Brown had many questions about his ventilator, and I went through the procedures from the hospital's parent training manual. Mrs. Brown understood the procedures and needed reassurance that she was doing things correctly. Mrs. Brown and I set up an another appointment for 2 weeks from today to talk about stimulating speech at home with the electrolarynx. Mrs. Brown is easy to talk with, and she tells me that she appreciates how we work as a team on Danny's speech program.

Danny at 20 Months

Danny responded well to his sign program during my treatment visit to his home. Mrs. Brown signs with us and has been able to incorporate signs into several routines during the day. Danny's older brother, Derek, 8, was there today, and he expressed an interest in reading to his brother after school each day. Derek seemed excited about learning signs for the vocabulary in two of Danny's favorite books. It is great that Derek now has a way to interact with his little brother.

Danny at 30 Months

I talked with Danny's respiratory therapist and surgeon today, and we agreed that Danny is now ready for a speaking valve. The order has been placed, and we will begin a speech stimulation program with the speaking valve as soon as possible. I can't wait to phone Mrs. Brown and tell her.

Danny at 4 Years

Danny is communicating with his speaking valve, using words clearly and combining words and signing. Our goal is to train use of some functional, short phrases.

Danny at 4½ Years

Speech, language, and cognitive testing has been completed with Danny over the past 4 months. I have shared the results with Mr. and Mrs. Brown, and they are pleased that Danny's cognitive skills are in the low average range on the *Kaufman Brief Intelligence Test for Children* and his receptive language skills were 2 months below age level on the *Preschool Language Scale-3*. His expressive language skills remain well below age level. The case manager will discuss school placement options for Danny with the Browns next week, and I will be there as well. I will consult with the speech-language pathologist at the school the Browns choose so that programs we have started will be continued.

SECTION

5

EVALUATING TREATMENT OUTCOMES AND DOCUMENTING SPEECH AND LANGUAGE CHARACTERISTICS OF CHILDREN WITH TRACHEOSTOMIES

BACKGROUND

There is a strong movement toward the implementation of evidence-based practice in many areas of rehabilitation science, including speech-language pathology. Logemann (2000) defines evidence-based practice as "using procedures that have been studied carefully and whose results have been reviewed and published", p. 3. She goes on to say that evidence-based practice "also takes into account current understanding of the pathophysiology of the disorder" (Logemann, 2000, p. 3). We have a way to go in the treatment of children with tracheostomies before we have a body of information about the best practices to employ with these children. Currently, the responsibility rests with those of us who work regularly with these children to:

1. Collect information systematically
2. Control for confounding factors when we conduct treatment
3. Watch for changes in the child that are greater than would be expected to occur because of maturation alone and/or for clinically meaningful change (Bain & Dollaghan, 1991; Logemann, 2000)

This section will highlight ways in which the speech-language pathologist can gather information to measure *outcomes* and *efficacy* of treatment for children with tracheostomies. Olswang (1998) defines and contrasts the differences between treatment outcomes and treatment efficacy. Treatment *outcomes* are ways of documenting a client's performance that show the benefits of treatment. The changes in a client's behavior make a difference to the client. Treatment *efficacy* is the documentation of evidence that the treatment has been effective and the clinician is confident that the changes are due to the treatment. The clinician has set up the treatment situation in such a way that she/he can rule out alternate explanations for the change in the client's behavior. In summary, changes can be shown when measuring both outcomes and efficacy, but measuring efficacy requires greater rigor in measurement and setting up the treatment goals so as to ensure that the treatment process most likely brought about the change in a client's behavior.

Measuring Treatment Outcomes and Goals

The documentation of the success of treatment with children with tracheostomies is in its infancy. There is shamefully little information about intervention with children with tracheostomies and about the ease or difficulty with which children have attained treatment goals. This section will suggest several ways that speech-language pathologists can start the documentation of treatment *outcomes*.

Adaptation to Wearing a Speaking Valve

Speech-language pathologists working with children who are about to have a speaking valve placed can document important information about the child's adaptation to the placement of a speaking valve (or occlusion of the stoma, or use of an electrolarynx, etc.)

MEASURES

1. Number of therapy sessions needed for the child to tolerate wearing the speaking valve for 5 minutes.
2. Number of therapy sessions needed for the child to tolerate wearing the speaking valve for 10 minutes.
3. Number of therapy sessions until the child vocalizes with the speaking valve for the first time.

PROCEDURES

Document the procedures used to place the valve, the type of valve worn by the child, the presence of a ventilator, pressure settings on the ventilator, and any other variables that may influence the child's adjustment to the speaking valve. The speech-language pathologist might want to follow standard procedures for placement of speaking valves outlined by Dikeman and Kazandjian (1995).

Effects or Outcomes of Vocal Stimulation

The outcomes of any vocal stimulation program can be measured with an assessment which will show changes in the child's level of vocalizations. For the child who uses primarily vowels, conducting inventories of the child's vowel use at periodic intervals may be most suitable. For children with more advanced vocalizations, a more complex analysis will be needed.

MEASURES

A number of measures may be used to document the outcome of vocal stimulation on the child's vocal output (See Section 3, "Intervention," for procedures for stimulating vocalizations):

1. Rate of vocalizations per minute produced by the child (included in Section 2, "Assessment")[a]
2. Child's inventory of vowels (included at the end of this section).
3. Child's inventory of consonants (included at the end of this section)
4. Ratio of consonant to vowel use (included in Section 2, "Assessment")
5. Syllable structure level or use of a higher percentage of syllables at a more complex level (move from using primarily vowels to use of CVs or VCs; included in Section 2, "Assessment").

PROCEDURES:

1. Use similar situations and procedures throughout the course of treatment.
2. Document the procedures that you use so that another speech-language pathologist can replicate what you have done.

[a]=The rate of vocalizing may be highly variable in children with tracheostomies (Morrison, 1998). Because the rate of vocalizing is highly variable, it is important to keep the situations and materials as consistent as possible. Additionally, the clinician should obtain an average of the vocalizations occurring in a series of observations rather than take a specific count in a set time.

3. The measures should be sensitive to small increments of change because children with tracheostomies will likely develop at a slower pace than children who are developing language normally. The measures listed above are sensitive to changes in developing children (Stoel-Gammon, 1992).

Measuring Treatment Efficacy/Use of a Single-Subject Design Procedure

Because children with tracheostomies are a highly heterogeneous group, one of the best ways to document changes in speech or language behaviors brought about by treatment is through use of single-subject design procedures whereby the child's progress in treatment is measured against his/her baseline performance prior to treatment.

Case Example

The following example will serve as a guide for speech-language pathologists who wish to document changes in a client's behavior due to treatment while ruling out changes due to extraneous factors or maturation. A multiple baseline design is employed. A child of 18 months with a tracheostomy and speaking valve newly in place was observed to communicate primarily through the use of vowels and consonant vowel syllables that contained a glottal plus a vowel. The child is comfortable with wearing the valve for periods of 20–30 minutes. The speech-language pathologist wished to set up a vocal stimulation program in which CVs or VCs containing early developing consonants were modeled for this child. Prior to beginning treatment, the speech-language pathologist followed these steps:

1. Selected a treatment goal and two control goals for the child.
2. Monitored the child's use of the treatment and control behaviors over a baseline period of 3 weeks, with two sessions per week.

   Target Goal: The child's spontaneous use of vocalizations were monitored to note the percentage of occurrence of CVs or VCs that contained true consonants (consonants other than the glottal stop or glottal fricative) during a 10-minute interaction with the speech-language pathologist while the child wore a speaking valve, over a 3-week period. Three measurements, one each week, were completed during the first session of the week. During this interaction, the child and speech-language pathologist played with some of the child's favorite toys.

   The number of CVs that occurred in 30 second intervals, with 30 seconds on, 30 seconds off, for a total of 10 intervals during a 10-minute period were calculated. The number of spontaneously produced CVs that occurred was divided by 10, and then multiplied by 100 to obtain a percentage of occurrence.

   The speech-language pathologist also administered a probe list of 10 VCs or CVs, which contained the same consonants as those trained, but the actual syllables would not be trained during treatment. The child was asked to spontaneously produce the CVs by naming the items or pictures representing the CVs on the list.

Control goals:

a. The percentage of occurrence of the spontaneous use of CVCs that occurred in a 10-minute interaction period between the clinician and child was noted.

(This goal may also serve as a generalization goal because the clinician might expect to see some transfer of the child's consonant use to the production of CVCs, but we would not expect a major change in this goal during the treatment and withdrawal phases).

b. The motor goal of making a circular drawing with a crayon on a page.

(This goal is unrelated to the target goal, is developmentally a 2 to 2½ year task, and is a task that the child has not been observed to complete. Therefore, we would not expect a change in performance).

3. Set up a treatment program for 5 weeks, two sessions per week.

Each treatment session started with a 10-minute free play session between the speech-language pathologist and the child. This play session was used for monitoring the goals for the child, then the probe list of untrained CVs and VCs was also administered.

The treatment consisted of a 10-minute interaction with the child, using common toys and objects or color pictures of familiar people. The clinician modeled the names of the toys, objects, or actions during three play routines that incorporated the objects. Eight target CVs or VCs were modeled: ball (ba), bye (bye), bee (bee), up (up), eat (eat), mom (ma), me (me), milk (mi). These are also common words appearing in the early lexicons of children developing language. For example, the clinician labeled a ball and pushed the ball back and forth with the child. At least five models of each CV or VC were presented. When the child pushed the ball back, the clinician prompted, "What do you do?" (waited for response). If no response occurred, the clinician modeled, "push ba."

4. Monitored the treatment and control goals for 3 weeks following treatment.

The probe list with nontrained CVs and VCs (and containing the target consonants) was administered once each week for 3 weeks following the treatment session. The spontaneous use of any CVs or VCs with true consonants in a 10-minute interaction with the speech-language pathologist was also noted.

The two control goals were also monitored following treatment. We might expect some change in the child's use of CVCs, but not in his/her scribbling a circle on a page. If the target goal changes during treatment while the other goals remain unchanged, the clinician can feel some confidence that the treatment brought about a change in the child's behaviors. The clinician also is interested in the child's performance on the target goal remaining fairly constant during the baseline period. If there were wide swings in performance, then the clinician would select another target for treatment. Several references are included in the "Resources" section that will provide the speech-language pathologist with excellent descriptions of single-subject designs (Frattali, 1998; McReynolds & Kearns, 1983).

LEARNING MORE ABOUT CHARACTERISTICS OF CHILDREN WITH TRACHEOSTOMIES

This section contains two suggestions for ways to document the speech and language characteristics of children with tracheostomies.

Documenting the Prevalence of Children with Tracheostomies

The number of tracheostomies that occur in the U.S. or in Canada in a given year or the number of children between 0–1 year, 1–2 years, and 2–3 years with tracheostomies is not clearly documented. Tracheostomy is a temporary condition compared to diagnosed syndromes (e.g., Down Syndrome) or medical conditions (e.g., cerebral palsy), and the placement of a tracheostomy generally occurs after, but not at birth. These issues may contribute to the difficulty in documenting the prevalence of children with tracheostomies. Yet we do know that the number of speech-language pathologists who encounter children with tracheostomies in place or with a history of tracheostomy has increased. Better documentation of the numbers of children likely to undergo tracheostomies would be useful in planning delivery of services for children with tracheostomies.

Procedure

Speech-language pathologists or physicians who work with children with tracheostomies on a regular basis in medical settings might document the following: (a) the number of live births within a specified period of time, and (b) through tracking patient numbers of the live births, follow the number of infants who then undergo tracheostomies within 3, 6, 9, or 12 months of the date of birth. A number of studies have documented the number of tracheostomies that occurred within a specified hospital setting within a year or 5 or 10 years. The missing piece is the denominator in the equation, or the percentage of the total population who underwent tracheostomies. Documentation of the total population from whom tracheostomized children were drawn would help researchers and clinicians to begin to document the prevalence of children with tracheostomies and to make comparisons between prevalence figures in different regions of the U.S. or Canada and between countries.

Documenting Speech and Language Characteristics

Because the number of children with tracheostomies that any one clinician or researcher will see is likely to remain small, speech-language pathologists who work with these children on a regular basis have an important role to play in documenting speech and language characteristics. The following are several suggestions that may be useful in documenting speech and language characteristics in children with tracheostomies.

Collection of Language Samples/Compilation of Language Samples Within a Database

1. Collect language samples containing at least 50 utterances.
2. Collect the sample within a semistructured free play situation and note the materials that were present in the room and the identity of the adult conversational partner (parent, clinician).

3. Follow the standard procedures for gathering language samples outlined by Miller (1981).

4. Transcribe the language sample, following rules for segmentation and inclusion of utterances outlined by Miller (1981).

5. Document the child's age, birthdate, opportunities afforded the child for vocalizing before and during cannulation, date and length of cannulation, whether the child was cannulated and whether a speaking valve was worn during elicitation of the sample, enrollment in speech and language therapy and any other pertinent information that would help describe the child and potential influences on speech and language development.

6. Take multiple samples over time, both during cannulation and after decannulation, using the same procedures each time.

7. Note changes in the child's mean length of utterance, the number of different words the child used, and progress in use of syntactic structures (noun phrase and verb phrase structures acquired in Brown's stages) (Miller, 1981).

   Once language samples have been gathered in a systematic manner, clinicians might consider placing them in a database such as the CHILDES database in order to provide a way for clinicians and researchers to access language information about children with tracheostomies (MacWhinney, 1989). Researchers could then access the transcripts and perform semantic and syntactic analyses, noting changes in a given child over time or productive language characteristics of children at given ages and of similar backgrounds.

Documentation of the Rate of Change in Speech Production Following Decannulation

Since we have longitudinal information regarding changes in speech production following decannulation on only a few children with tracheostomies, careful documentation of changes in children following decannulation by speech-language pathologists during this time would be extremely useful. Use of measures that have been shown to document changes in several children with tracheostomies is advocated (Locke & Pearson, 1990; Bleile, 1998).

PROCEDURES

1. Document information about the child's age, receptive language skills, and vocabulary size that corresponds to each of the measurements below.

2. Based on speech samples (preferably at least 20 utterances), note the size and content of the child's phonetic inventory (See Section 2, "Assessment").

3. Based on speech samples (preferably at least 50 utterances), count the number of syllables that contain a true consonant and divide by the total number of utterances. Calculate the percentage of canonical syllables produced by the child (see Section 2, "Assessment").

4. Take measurements frequently (once a month, when possible).

5. By following the rate of change in number and types of consonants added to the inventory and the length of time needed for the child to reach a canonical babbling stage, the speech-language pathologist can begin to predict the rate of change experienced by children following tracheostomies.

PROCEDURES AND FORMS USED TO MONITOR CHANGE

The following section contains additional forms the speech-language pathologist will want to use in documenting changes in children who have tracheostomies.

Form 5–1. Vowel Matrix

Child: ____________________ Date: ____________________

Vowel Matrix

Front	Mid High	Back
i beat		u boot
I bit		U book
e bate	ɝ Bert	o boat
ɛ bet	ɚ ə ^ butter, again, but	ɔ bought
ae bat		a bomb

Low

Circle vowels that the child is observed to use.

Form 5–2. Consonant Inventories (Initial, Medial, Final)

Child: ________________

Date: ____________________

Sample Size/ Characteristics: ____________________

Manner	***Place***	***Voiced***	***Voiceless***
Nasals	Bilabial	m	
	Alveolar	n	
	Velar	ŋ (M,F)[a]	
Stops	Bilabial	b	p
	Alveolar	d	t
	Velar	g	k
	Glottal	? (M,F)	
Glides	Labial	w	ʍ
	Velar	j	
Fricatives	Labiodental	v	f
	Linguadental	ð	θ
	Alveolar	z	s
	Palatal	ʒ	ʃ
	Glottal	h	
Affricates	Palatal	dʒ	tʃ
Liquids	Alveolar	l	
Palatal		r (I, M)	

Circle consonants that the child uses in each position in two different words (Stoel-Gammon, 1985).

[a] = Sound occurs in these positions only.

Form 5–3. Syllable Shape Chart

Child: ______________________ Date: ____________________

Shape	*Number of Occurrences*	*Number of Opportunities*
V		
CV		
VC		
CVCV		
CVC		
CCV		
VCC		
CCVC		
CVCC		
CCCV		
CCCVC		

This chart may be used as an intermediate step when calculating syllable structure level.

Form 5–4. Summary of Phonological Process Use

Child: ______________________ Date: ______________________

Phonological Processes	***Number of Occurrences***	***Possible Occurrences***	***Percentage of Occurrences***
Phonological			
Omissions			
Syllable Reduction			
Consonant Sequence			
Reduction			
Prevocalic Consonant			
Omissions			
Postvocalic Consonant			
Omissions			
Class Deficiencies			
Stridents			
Velar Obstruents			
Liquid L			
Liquid R			
Nasals			
Glides			

Note. Based on phonological processes assessed with the Assessment of Phonological Processes-Revised (Hodson, 1986). Reprinted with permission of Pro-Ed, Inc., Austin, TX.

GLOSSARY

Airway Obstruction: a blockage of the trachea that results from congenital, structural irregularities or from a collapsing of the tissue and makes the passage of air difficult or impossible.

Anomalies: structural or anatomical irregularities of the head or neck that influence respiratory functioning or that block the free flow of air.

Aspiration: the entry of fluids or foreign particles (food, saliva) below the laryngeal area into the bronchial passages and lungs.

Brain Hemorrhage: bleeding in the brain that may result if medically fragile children are overstimulated and become distressed.

Bronchopulmonary Dysplasia: chronic lung condition resulting from prematurity or from trauma to the lungs resulting from adverse effects of mechanical ventilation.

Central Hypoventricular Syndrome: a congenital problem with the central nervous system mechanism that stimulates breathing while a child sleeps and results in the inability to breathe spontaneously while asleep.

Cerebral Palsy: a nonprogressive, but permanent neuromuscular impairment resulting from difficulties in early brain development. The disease most commonly results in the child having difficulty controlling muscle movements and posture as well as abnormalities in muscle tone.

Chronicity: the length of time from birth until the medical condition is resolved.

Conventional: verbalizations or gestures that signal a specific meaning or function and that are easily understood. Conventional gestures include giving or pointing. Conventional verbalizations include words or phonetically consistent forms.

Cuffed tracheostomy: a balloon mechanism that can be inflated on the distal end of the tracheal tube to create a seal in the trachea.

Deictic gestures: gestures that indicate or refer to an object or person, e.g., showing, pointing, giving, and reaching (Iverson & Thal, 1998).

Duchennes Muscular Dystrophy: an X-linked neuromuscular disease that results in progressive muscle weakness, with many patients confined to wheelchairs by 7 to 12 years of age. Complications may include progressive respiratory muscle weakness requiring mechanical ventilation and tracheostomy as the disease progresses. Lung infections, swallowing complications, and airway obstructions may occur.

Eye gaze: gaze directed at an adult's face. Children use shifts in eye gaze from person to object and back to person to establish reference (Wetherby & Prizant, 1993).

Granulation: tissue that forms at the site of the stoma in response to a tracheostomy tube that is in place.

Hypoxia: limitation in the amount of oxygen reaching the tissues.

Intentions: the reasons for, or functions of communication. Early intentions include requesting, commenting, and rejecting, prior to the onset of the use of words (Wetherby, Cain, Yonclas, & Walker, 1988).

Intentional: the child interacts in a way that is deliberate to gain the attention of an adult (Bates, Camaioni, & Volterra, 1975).

Intubation: placement of a tube either in the nose or the mouth and then through the trachea so that air can reach the lungs and/or the airway can be cleared of fluids.

Joint attention: the child and a partner both attend to the same object or person. Joint attention serves to establish a referent or topic of interaction or conversation. One partner may point to direct the other's attention to an object or event.

Lax vowels: vowels produced with less muscle activity and that are usually shorter in length, e.g., [ae] or [U].

Low birth weight: defined as a weight of 2,500 grams or less at birth. Two categories of low birth weight exist: (a) infants born before 37 weeks gestation, and (b) infants born at term who are small for gestational age.

Mechanical ventilator: the mechanical equipment that pumps air in and out of the lungs and helps to maintain airflow when a child's breathing cannot maintain an adequate air supply.

Oximeter: a noninvasive device that is used to measure the oxygen saturation in the blood and carbon dioxide levels.

Oxygen concentration, or FIO_2: the concentration of inspired oxygen from a ventilator. This concentration is measured in decimals, where .80 is an 80% concentration of oxygen. This level is ideally .40 to wean a patient from a ventilator.

Peak Inspiratory Pressure, or PIP: the peak of pressure during inspiration, both PIP and PEEP are measured or preset on ventilators.

Positive End Expiratory Pressure, or PEEP: the amount of air that stays in the lungs at the end of a full expiration; a speaking valve may increase the level of PEEP.

Prematurity: the birth of a child prior to full term of $\leq$ 37 weeks and weighing less than 2,500 grams.

Rate of respiration: usually measured as the ratio of inspiration to expiration, the flow rate determines the length of inspiration. The rate of expiration is usually 1.5 times the length of inspiration. When the flow rate is decreased, a patient has longer to talk on expiration.

Recognitory: a gesture in which the function of an object is depicted through action completed with the object or an empty word (e.g., pretending to eat with a fork) (Thal & Bates, 1988).

Representational gestures: gestures that establish reference as well as carry a specific semantic content. They include the categories of object related (e.g., drinking from a cup or same motion with an empty hand) and culturally defined conventional gestures (e.g., waving bye-bye) (Iverson & Thal, 1998, p. 61).

Respiratory distress syndrome: a condition in which the lungs become overexpanded and the result is ineffective or labored breathing.

Severity: length of time children with chronic health problems spend in the hospital to resolve the condition(s).

Small for gestational age: used to "refer to an infant whose birth weight is at the 10th percentile or less of the expected weight for their gestational age" (Gallagher & Watkin, 1998, p. 18).

Stoma: the opening in the neck that is created when the tracheotomy is performed.

Technologically dependent: child who needs both a medical device to compensate for the loss of a vital bodily function and substantial and ongoing nursing care to avert death or further disability (U.S. Congress, 1987, p. 3).

Tracheostomy tube or cannula: the plastic or metal tube that is inserted into the trachea at the time of a tracheotomy to keep the airway open.

Tracheomalacia: a weakening or collapse of the tracheal cartilage that may result in the obstruction of the airway.

Ventilator mode: refers to how the air is delivered to the patient and the amount of breathing the patient will do on his/her own. SIMV, or synchronized intermittent mandatory ventilation, uses the child's inspiration to trigger the ventilator.

Vocal cord paralysis: an inability to move one or both vocal cords due to nerve damage or physical trauma.

RESOURCES

RESOURCES FOR SECTIONS 1–5

Resources listed here support the topics discussed in Sections 1–5.

American Speech and Hearing Association (1996). User's Guide: Phase I-Group III. National Treatment Outcome Data Collection Project. Task Force on Treatment Outcome/Cost Effectiveness. Rockville, MD: American Speech and Hearing Association.

American Speech-Language-Hearing Association (1998). Managing communication and swallowing impairments in tracheostomized and ventilator-dependent adults. Videoconference. Videotape and materials available from ASHA, 10801 Rockville Pike, Rockville, MD, 20852-3279.

Arvedson, J. C., & Brodsky, L. (1993). *Pediatric swallowing and feeding: Assessment and management.* San Diego, CA: Singular Publishing Group.

Bain, B., & Dollaghan, C. (1991). Clinical Forum: Treatment efficacy: The notion of clinically significant change. *Language, Speech and Hearing Services in Schools, 22*, 264–270.

Bendersky, M., & Lewis, M. (1994). Environmental risk, biological risk, and developmental outcome. *Developmental Psychology, 30*(4), 484–494.

Berman, S. S. (1996). *Phonology for groups: Thematic activities for everyday settings.* San Antonio, TX: Communication Skill Builders.

Bivonia Medical Technologies, Inc., 5700 West 23rd Avenue, Gary, IN, 46406, 1-800-348-6064.

Boston Medical Products, 117 Flanders Road, Westborough, MA, 01581.

Chapman, R. S. (1981). Exploring children's communicative intents. In J. Miller (Ed.), *Assessing language production in children.* (pp. 111–138). Baltimore: University Park Press.

Dikeman, K. J., & Kazandjian, M. S. (1995). Oral communication options. In K. Dikeman and M. Kazandjian (Eds.), *Communication and swallowing management of tracheostomized and ventilator-dependent adults.* (pp. 141–196). San Diego, CA: Singular Publishing Group.

Hodson, B. W., & Paden, E. P. (1991). *Targeting intelligible speech: A phonological approach to remediation. 2nd Ed.* San Diego, CA: College Hill Press.

Hood Laboratories, 575 Washington Street, Pembroke, MA, 02359.

Kaufman, A., & Kaufman, N. (1983). *Kaufman Assessment Battery For Children.* Circle Pines, MN: American Guidance Service.

Kennedy, A. H., Johnson, N. G., & Sturdevant, E. W. (1982). An educational program for families of children with tracheostomies. *American Journal of Maternal-Child Nursing*, 42–49.

Kersten, L. D. (1989). Tracheostomy and tracheostomy tubes. In L. D. Kersten (Ed.), *Comprehensive respiratory nursing. A decision making approach.* (pp. 652–699). Toronto, ON: W. B. Saunders Co.

Kersten, L. D. (1989). Mechanical ventilation. In L. D. Kersten (Ed.), *Comprehensive respiratory nursing. A decision making approach.* (pp. 700–750). Toronto, ON: W. B. Saunders Co.

King, S., Kertoy, M., King, G., Rosenbaum, P., Hurley, P., & Law, M. (2000). Children with disabilities in Ontario: A profile of children's services. Part 2: Perceptions about family-centred service delivery for children with disabilities. CanChild Centre for Childhood Disability Research, McMaster University, Hamilton, Ontario, June, 2000.

Law, M. (1998). Special issue: Family centred assessment and intervention in pediatric rehabilitation. *Physical and Occupational Therapy in Pediatrics, 18*(1), 1–102.

Lowe, M., & Costello, A. (1976). *Manual for the symbolic play test.* London: NFER-Nelson.

MacWhinney, B. (1989). *Child language analysis.* Manual for use of the CLAN programs for the Child Language Data Exchange. Dept. of Psychology, Carnegie Mellon University, Pittsburgh, PA, 15213. Child Language Data Exchange, *http://poppy.psy.cmu.edu/childes/index.html*

Mallinckrodt Medical, Inc., 675 McDonnell Blvd. P. O. Box 5840, Hazelwood, MO, 63434, 1-888-744-1414.

Mason, M., & Watkins, C. (1992). Protocol for the use of the Passy-Muir tracheostomy speaking valves. *The European Respiratory Journal, 5*(15), 148.

McReynolds, L. V., & Kearns, K. P. (1983). *Single-subject experimental designs in communicative disorders.* Baltimore, MD: University Park Press.

McWilliam, P. J., Winton, P. J., & Crais, E. R. (1996). *Practical strategies for family-centered intervention.* San Diego, CA: Singular Publishing Group, Inc.

Miller, J. F. (1981). *Assessing language production in children: Experimental procedures.* Boston, MA: Allyn and Bacon.

Nellcor Puritan Bennett, 4280 Hacienda Drive, Pleasanton, California, 94588.

Owens, R. E. (1999). Specific intervention techniques. In R. E. Owens (Ed.), *Language disorders: A functional approach to assessment and intervention.* (pp. 285–360). Boston, MA: Allyn and Bacon.

Passy-Muir, Inc. (1998). Educational seminar videotape and manual. Available from Passy Muir Inc., 4521 Campus Drive, Suite 273, Irvine, CA 92715. 1-800-634-5397.

Paul, R. (1995). Appendix 10-1. Children's books that employ semantic and syntactic patterns commonly targeted in language intervention. In R. Paul (Ed.), *Language disorders from infancy through adolescence: Assessment and intervention.* (pp. 360–365). St. Louis, MO: Mosby.

Pilling Weck, 420 Delaware Drive, Fort Washington, PA, 19034. 1-800-523-6507.

Rathlev, M. C., & McNamara, M. A. (1982). Teaching families to give trach care at home. *Nursing, 11*(6), 81–82.

Rosin, P., Whitehead, A., Tuchman, L., Jesien, G., Begun, A., & Irwin, L. (1996). *Partnerships in family-centered care: A guide to collaborative early intervention.* Baltimore, MD: Paul H. Brookes Publishing Co.

Secord, W. (1985). The traditional approach to articulation treatment. In P. Newman, N. Creaghead, and W. Secord (Eds.), *Assessment and remediation of articulation and phonological disorders.* (pp. 127–158). Columbus, OH: Merrill Publishing.

Steifel, G., Plunkett, J., & Meisels, S. (1987). Affective expression among preterm infants of varying levels of biological risk. *Infant Behavior and Development, 10,* 151–164.

Tippet, D. (2000). *Tracheostomy and ventilator dependency: Management of breathing, speaking and swallowing.* New York: Thieme Medical Publishers, Inc.

VandenBerg, K. A. (1993). Basic competencies to begin developmental care in the intensive care nursery. *Infants and Young Children, 6*(2), 52–59.

RESOURCES ON TRACHEOSTOMY ORGANIZED BY TOPIC

Resources listed here were selected from a large medical reference database based on their usefulness for speech-language pathologists.

Pierre Robin Syndrome

Augarten, A., Sagy, M., Yahav, J., & Barsilay, Z. (1990). Management of upper airway obstruction in the Pierre Robin syndrome. *British Journal of Oral Maxillofacial Surgery, 28*(2), 105–108.

Bath, A., & Bull, P. (1997). Management of upper airway obstruction in Pierre Robin sequence. *Journal of Laryngology and Otolology, 111*(12), 1155–1157.

Caouette-Laberge, L., Bayet, B., & Larocque, Y. (1994). The Pierre Robin sequence: Review of 125 cases and evolution of treatment modalities. *Plastic and Reconstructive Surgery, 93*(5), 934–942.

Dudkiewicz, Z., Sekula, E., & Nielepiec-Jalosinska, A. (2000). Gastroesophageal reflux in Pierre Robin sequence—Early treatment. *Cleft Palate-Craniofacial Journal, 37*(2), 205–208.

Bronchopulmonary Dysplasia

Ariagno, R., Fulroth, R., Baldwin, R., & Glotzbach, S. (1991). Incidence of bronchopulmonary dysplasia, growth failure, and pulmonary dysfunction assessed by clinical scoring. *Journal of Perinatology, 11*(4), 311–314.

Barrington, K., & Finer, N. (1998). Treatment of bronchopulmonary dysplasia: A review. *Clinics in Perinatology, 25*(1), 177–202.

Gregoire, M., Lefebvre, F., & Glorieux, J. (1998). Health and development outcomes at 18 months in very preterm infants with bronchopulmonary dysplasia. *Pediatrics, 101*(5), 856–860.

Katz, R., & McWilliams, B. (1988). Bronchopulmonary dysplasia in the pediatric intensive care unit. *Critical Care Clinics, 4*(4), 755–787.

Martin, R., & Pridham, K. (1992). Early experiences of parents feeding their infants with bronchopulmonary dysplasia. *Neonatal Network, 11*(3), 23–29.

Martin, R., & Walsh-Sukys, M. (1999). Bronchopulmonary dysplasia—no simple solution. *New England Journal of Medicine, 340*(13), 1036–1038.

Tahy, A., McMullen, E., & Kim, S. (1988). Later growth and development in premature infants with Bronchopulmonary Dysplasia (BPD). *Journal of Pediatric and Perinatal Nutrition, 2*(1), 67–77.

Tracheomalacia

Beasley, S., & Qi, B. (1998). Understanding tracheomalacia. *Journal of Pediatrics and Child Health, 34*(3), 209–210.

Cacciaguerra, S., & Bianchi, A. (1998). Tracheal ring-graft reinforcement in lieu of tracheostomy for tracheomalacia. *Pediatric Surgery International, 13*(8), 556–559.

Callahan, C. (1998). Primary tracheomalacia and gastroesophageal reflux in infants with cough. *Clinical Pediatrics, 37*(12), 725–731.

Davis, S., Jones, M., Kisling, J., Angelicchio, C., & Tepper, R. (1998). Effect of continuous positive pressure on forced expiratory flows in infants with tracheomalacia. *American Journal of Respiratory and Critical Care Medicine, 158*(1), 148–152.

Doull, I., Mok, Q., & Tasker, R. (1997). Tracheomalacia in preterm infants with chronic lung disease. *Archives of Disease in Childhood. Fetal and Neonatal Edition, 76*(3), 203–205.

Furman, R., Backer, C., Dunham, M., Donaldson, J., Mavroudis, C., & Holinger, L. (1999). The use of balloon-expandable metallic stents in the treatment of pediatric tracheomalacia and bronchomalacia. *Archives of Otolaryngology—Head and Neck Surgery, 125*(2), 203–207.

Hypoventilation Syndrome

Gozal, D., & Harper, R. (1999). Novel insights into congenital hypoventilation syndrome. *Current Opinion in Pulmonary Medicine, 5*(6), 335–338.

Gozal, D. Marcus, C., Shoseyov, D., & Keens, T. (1993). Peripheral chemoreceptor function in children with the congenital central hypoventilation syndrome. *Journal of Applied Physiology, 74*(1), 379–387.

Katz, E., McGrath, S., & Marcus, C. (2000). Late-onset central hypoventilation with hypothalamic dysfunction: A distinct clinical syndrome. *Pediatric Pulmonology, 29*(1), 62–68.

Marcus, C., Jansen, M., Poulsen, M., Keens, S., Nield, T., Lipsker, L., & Keens, T. (1991). Medical and psychosocial outcome of children with congenital central hypoventilation syndrome. *Journal of Pediatrics, 119*(6), 888–895.

Oren, J., Kelly, D., & Shannon, D. (1987). Long-term follow-up of children with congenital central hypoventilation syndrome. *Pediatrics, 80*(3), 375–380.

Silvestri, J., Weese-Mayer, D., & Nelson, M. (1992). Neuropsychological abnormalities in children with congenital central hypoventilation syndrome. *Journal of Pediatrics, 120*(3), 388–393.

Strauser, L., Helikson, M., & Tobias, J. (1999). Anesthetic care for the child with congenital central alveolar hypoventilation syndrome (Ondine's curse). *Journal of Clinical Anesthesia, 11*(5), 431–437.

Weese-Mayer, D., Silvestri, J., Menzies, L., Morrow-Kenny, A., Hunt, C., & Hauptman, S. (1992). Congenital central hypoventilation syndrome: Diagnosis, management, and long-term outcome in thirty-two children. *Journal of Pediatrics, 120*(3), 381–387.

Burn Patients

Barret, J., Desai, M., & Herndon, D. (2000). Effects of tracheostomies on infection and airway complications in pediatric burn patients. *Burns, 26*(2), 190–193.

Coln, C. Purdue, G., & Hunt, J. (1998). Tracheostomy in the young pediatric burn patient. *Archive of Surgery, 133*(5), 537–540.

Hunt, J., Purdue, G., & Gunning, T. (1986). Is tracheostomy warranted in the burn patient? Indications and complications. *Journal of Burn Care and Rehabilitation, 7*(6), 492–495.

Jones, W., Madden, M., Finkelstein, J., Yurt, R., & Goodwin, C. (1989). Tracheostomies in burn patients. *Annals of Surgery, 209*(4), 471–474.

Rodeberg, D., Maschinot, N., Housinger, T., & Warden, G. (1992). Decreased pulmonary barotrauma with the use of volumetric diffusive respiration in pediatric patients with burns: The 1992 Moyer Award. *Journal of Burn Care and Rehabilitation, 13*(5), 506–511.

Venus, B., Matsuda, T., Copiozo, J., & Mathru, M. (1981). Prophylactic intubation and continuous positive airway pressure in the management of inhalation injury in burn victims. *Critical Care Medicine, 9*(7), 519–523.

Yang, J., Yang, W., Chang, L., & Chuang, S. (1999). Symptomatic tracheal stenosis in burns. *Burns, 25*(1), 72–80.

Whitelock-Jones, L., Bass, D., Millar, A., & Rode, H. (1999). Inhalation burns in children. *Pediatric Surgery International, 15*(1), 50–55.

Airway Obstruction

Altman, K., Wetmore, R., & Marsh. (1997). Congenital airway abnormalities requiring tracheotomy: A profile of 56 patients and their diagnoses over a 9 year period. *International Journal of Pediatric Otorhinolaryngology, 41*(2), 199–206.

Choi, S., & Zalzal, G. (2000). Changing trends in neonatal subglottic stenosis. *Otolaryngology—Head and Neck Surgery, 122*(1), 61–63.

Cotton, R. (2000). Management of subglottic stenosis. *Otolaryngologic Clinics of North America, 33*(1), 111–130.

Liu, J., Hartnick, C., Rutter, M., Hartley, B., & Myer, C. (2000). Subglottic stenosis associated with transesophageal echocardiography. *International Journal of Pediatric Otorhinolaryngology, 55*(1), 47–49.

Massie, R., Robertson, C., & Berkowitz, R. (2000). Long-term outcome of surgically treated acquired subglottic stenosis in infancy. *Pediatric Pulmonology, 30*(2), 125–130.

Meneghini, L., Zadra, N., Metrangolo, S., Narne, S., & Giusti, F. (2000). Post-intubation subglottal stenosis in children: Risk factors and prevention in pediatric intensive care. *Minerva Anestesiologica, 66*(6), 467–471.

Vollrath, M., Freihorst, J., & von der Hardt, H. (1999). Surgery of acquired laryngotracheal stenosis in childhood. Experiences and results from 1988 to 1998. I: Laryngotracheal reconstruction. *HNO, 47*(5), 457–465.

Walner, D., & Holinger, L. (1997). Supraglottic stenosis in infants and children. A preliminary report. *Archive of Otolaryngology—Head and Neck Surgery, 123*(3), 337–341.

Laryngotracheal Trauma

Kadish, H., Schunk, J., & Woodward, G. (1994). Blunt pediatric laryngotracheal trauma: Case reports and review of the literature. *American Journal of Emergency Medicine, 12*(2), 207–211.

Recurrent Respiratory Papilomatosis

Armstrong, L., Derkay, C., & Reeves, W. (1999). Initial results from the national registry for juvenile-onset recurrent respiratory Papilomatosis. RRP Task Force. *Archives of Otolaryngology—Head and Neck Surgery, 125*(7), 743–748.

Berkowitz, R. (1995). Pediatric laryngotracheal reconstruction: Melbourne experiment at the Royal Children's Hospital. *Australian and New Zealand Journal of Surgery, 65*(9), 650–653.

Prevalence of Tracheostomy in Children

Donelly, M., Lacey, P., & Maguire, A. (1996). A twenty year (1971–1990) review of tracheostomies in a major pediatric hospital. *International Journal of Otorhinolaryngology, 35*(1), 1–9.

Dubey, S.P., & Garap, J. P. (1999). Pediatric tracheostomy: An analysis of 40 cases. *Journal of Laryngology and Otology, 113*(7), 645–651.

Palfrey, J., Hayine, M., Porter, S., Fenton, T., Cooperman-Vincent, P., Shaw, D., Johnson, B., Bierle, T., & Walker, D. (1994). Prevalence of medical technology assistance among children in Massachusetts in 1987 and 1990. *Public Health Report, 109*(2), 226–233.

Sakakihara, Y., Yoneyama, A., & Kamoshita, S. (1993). Chronic ventilator-assisted children in university hospitals in Japan. *Acta Paediatrica Japonica, 35*(4), 332–335.

Speech and Tracheostomy

American Speech and Hearing Association. (1998). Speech for patients with tracheostomies or ventilators. *American Speech and Hearing Association, 40*(1), 37–38.

Bell, S. (1996). Use of Passy-Muir tracheostomy speaking valve in mechanically-dependent neurological patients. *Critical Care Nurse, 16*(1), 63–68.

Kaut, K., Turcott, J., & Lavery, M. (1996). Passy-Muir speaking valve. *Dimensions of Critical Care Nursing, 15*(6), 298–306.

Leder, S. (1994). Perceptual rankings of speech quality produced with one-way tracheostomy speaking valves. *Journal of Speech and Hearing Research, 37*(6), 1308–1312.

Speech in Children with Tracheostomies

Fraser, J., Pengilly, A., & Mok, Q. (1998). Long-term ventilator-dependent children: A vocal profile analysis. *Pediatric Rehabilitation, 2*(2), 71–75.

Handler, S., Simon, B., & Fowler, S. (1983) Speech and the child with long-term tracheostomy—the problem and the otolaryngologist's role. *Otolaryngology—Head and Neck Surgery, 92*(6), 625–627.

Jackson, D., & Albamonte, S. (1994). Enhancing communication with the Passy-Muir valve. *Pediatric Nursing, 20*(2), 149–153.

Kaslon, K., & Stein, R. (1985). Chronic pediatric tracheotomy: Assessment and implications for habilitation of voice, speech and language in young children. *International Journal of Pediatric Otorhinolaryngology, 9,* 165–171.

Simon, B., & Handler, S. (1981). The speech pathologist and management of children with tracheostomies. *Journal of Otolaryngology, 10*(6), 440–448.

Yagani, N., Tanigami, H., Watanabe, Y., & Kumon, K. (1995). A problem with an infant speaking tracheostomy tube. *Anesthesia, 50*(1), 91–92.

Speech in Adults with Tracheostomies

Elichar, I. (2000). Unaided speech in long-term tube-free tracheostomy. *Laryngoscope, 110*(5 pt 1), 749–760.

King, S. (1994). The tracheotomized patient: Tracheal toilet and speech. *Clinical Pulmonary Medicine, 1*(6), 365–368.

Zajac, D., Fornataro-Clerici, L., & Roop, T. (1999). Aerodynamic characteristics of tracheostomy speaking valves: An updated report. *Journal of Speech and Hearing Research, 42*(1), 92–100.

Parent's Perceptions and Concerns

Bach, J. (1993). A comparison of long-term ventilatory support alternatives from the perspective of the patient and caregiver. *Chest, 104*(6), 1702–1706.

Bahng, S., VanHala, S., Nelson, V., Hurvitz, E., Roloff, D., Grady, E., & Lewis, C. (1998). Parental report of pediatric tracheostomy care. *Archive of Physical Medicine and Rehabilitation, 79*(11), 1367–1369.

Baumgardner, D., & Burtea, E. (1998). Quality-of-life in technology-dependent children receiving homecare, and their families—a qualitative study. *Wisconsin Medical Journal, 97*(8), 51–55.

Cohen, S., Suzman, K., Simms, C., Burstein, F., Riski, J., & Montgomery, G. (1998). Sleep apnea surgery versus tracheostomy in children: An exploratory study of the comparative effects on quality of life. *Plastic and Reconstructive Surgery, 102*(6), 1855–1864.

Gilinson, P. (1988). Acquired subglottic stenosis in infants. The parent's view. *Journal of Laryngology and Otology. Supplement, 17,* 41–44.

Kun, S., & Warburton, D. (1987). Telephone assessment of parents' knowledge of home-care treatments and readmission outcomes for high-risk infants and toddlers. *American Journal of Diseases of Children, 141*(8), 888–892.

Pizzuto, M., Volk, M., & Kingston, L. (1998). Common topics in pediatric otolaryngology. *Pediatric Clinics of North America, 45*(4), 973–991.

Shintani, T., Asakura, K., Ishi, K., Yoshida, M., Kataura, A., & Ogasawara, H. (1998). Obstructive sleep apnea in children with cerebral palsy. *Nippon Jibiinkoka Gakkai Kaiho [Journal of the Oto-Rhino-Laryngological Society of Japan], 101*(3), 266–271.

Turnage, C., & Engleman, S. (1994). Discharge education for parents of infants with tracheostomies. *Journal of Pediatric Nursing, 9*(6), 425–426.

Wills, J. (1983). Concerns and needs of mothers providing home care for children with tracheostomies. *Maternal-Child Nursing Journal, 12*(2), 89–107.

Early Care, Intensive Care, and Tracheostomy

deBoisblanc, M., Goldman, R., Mayberry, J., Brand, D., Pangburn, P., Soifer, B., & Mullins, R. (2000). Weaning injured patients with prolonged pulmonary failure from mechanical ventilation in a non-intensive care unit setting. *Journal of Trauma, 49*(2), 224–230.

Godwin, J., & Heffner, J. (1991). Special considerations in tracheostomy management. *Clinical Chest Medicine, 12*(3), 573–583.

Kollef, M., Ahrens, T., & Shannon, W. (1999). Clinical predictors and outcomes for patients requiring tracheostomy in the intensive care unit. *Critical Care Medicine, 27*(9), 1714–1720.

Schwerdt, M. (1996). Growing up on the intensive care unit. Results of a survey on quality of life of long-term ventilated children on intensive care units. *Med Klinik, 91*(Suppl. 2), 53–55.

Senders, C., Muntz, H., & Schweiss, D. (1991). Physician survey on the care of children with tracheotomy. *American Journal of Otolaryngology, 12*(1), 48–50.

Shneerson, J. (1996). Home mechanical ventilation in children: Techniques, outcomes and ethics. *Monaldi Archives for Chest Disease, 51*(5), 426–430.

Slonim, A., Patel, K., Ruttiman, U., & Pollack, M. (2000). The impact of prematurity: A perspective of pediatric intensive care units. *Critical Care Medicine, 28*(3), 848–853.

Stott, S. (2000). Recent advances: Recent advances in intensive care. *British Medical Journal, 320*(7231), 358–361.

Feeding Problems and Tracheostomy

Bath, A., & Bull, P. (1997). Management of upper airway obstruction in Pierre Robin Sequence. *Journal of Laryngology and Otology, 111*(12), 1155–1157.

Bauer, M., & Lyrene, R. (1999). Chronic aspiration in children: Evaluation of the lipid-laden macrophage index. *Pediatric Pulmonology, 28*(2), 94–100.

Hansen, H., & Jorgensen, S. (1968). Tracheostomy and prolonged nasotrachial intubation. *Danish Medical Bulletin, 15*(2), 53–57.

Huerta, G., & Puri, V. (2000). Nasoenteric feeding tubes in critically ill patients (fluroscopy versus blind). *Nutrition, 16*(4), 264–267.

Mackay, L., Morgan, A., & Berstein, B. (1999). Swallowing disorders in severe brain injury: Risk factors affecting return to oral intake. *Archive of Physical Medicine and Rehabilitation, 80*(4), 365–371.

Prodoehl, D., & Shattuck, K. (1995). Nasogastric intubation for nutrition and airway protection in infants with Pierre Robin sequence. *Journal of Perinatology, 15*(5), 395–397.

Schnapf, B., Favrot, J., & Dodson, S. (1993). Esophageal obstruction in a tracheotomized infant. *Chest, 104*(6), 1909–1910.

Singer, L., & Sidoti, E. (1992). Pediatric management of robin sequence. *Cleft Palate-Craniofacial Journal, 29*(3), 220–223.

Strauss, D., Kastner, T., Ashwal, S., & White, J. (1997). Tube feeding and mortality in children with severe disability and mental retardation. *Pediatrics, 99*(3), 358–362.

Willging, J. (2000). Benefit of feeding assessment before pediatric airway reconstruction. *Laryngoscope, 110*(5 pt. 1), 825–834.

Medical Outcomes and Complications of Tracheostomy

Buschbacher, R. (1995). Outcomes and problems in pediatric pulmonary rehabilitation. *American Journal of Physical Medicine and Rehabilitation, 74*(4), 287–293.

Dubey, S., & Garap, J. (1999). Pediatric tracheostomy: An analysis of 40 cases. *Journal of Laryngology and Otology, 113*(7), 645–651.

Gluth, M., Maska, S., Nelson, J., & Otto, R. (2000). Postoperative management of pediatric tracheostomy: Results of nationwide survey. *Otolaryngology—Head and Neck Surgery, 122*(5), 701–705.

Gregoire, M., Lefebvre, F., & Glorieux, J. (1998). Health and development outcomes at 18 months in very preterm infants with bronchopulmonary dysplasia. *Pediatrics, 101*(5), 856–860.

Jardine, E., O'Toole, M., Paton, J., & Wallis, C. (1999). Current status of long-term ventilation in the United Kingdom: Questionnaire survey. *British Medical Journal, 318*(7179), 295–299.

Kleinsasser, N., Merkenschlager, A., Schroter, C., Mattick, C., Nicolai, T., & Mantel, K. (1996). Fatal complications in tracheotomized children. *Laryngo-Rhino-Otologie, 75*(2), 77–82.

Kurek, C., Cohen, I., Lambrinos, J., Minatoya, K., Booth, F., & Chalfin, D. (1997). Clinical and economic outcome of patients undergoing tracheostomy for prolonged mechanical ventilation in New York state during 1993: Analysis of 6,353 cases under diagnosis-related group 483. *Critical Care Medicine, 25*(6), 983–988.

Orlowski, J., Ellis, N., Amin, N., & Crumrine, R. (1980). Complications of airway intrusion in 100 consecutive cases in pediatric ICU. *Critical Care Medicine, 8*(6), 324–331.

Schlessel, J., Harper, R., Rappa, H., Kenigsber, K., & Khanna, S. (1993). Tracheostomy: Acute and long-term mortality and morbidity in very low birth weight premature infants. *Journal of Pediatric Surgery, 28*(7), 873–876.

Schwerdt, M. (1996). Growing up on the intensive care unit. Results of a survey of quality of life of long-term ventilated children on intensive care units. *Med Klinik, 12*(91), Suppl. 2, 53–55.

Swift, A., & Rogers, J. (1987). The changing indications for tracheostomy in children. *Journal of Laryngology and Otology, 101*(12), 1258–1262.

Mechanical Ventilation

Armstrong, R., Bullen, C., Cohen, S., Singer, M., & Webb, A. (1992). Intermittent positive ventilation. *Clinical Intensive Care, 3*(4), 190.

Brook, A., Ahrens, T., Schaiff, R., Prentice, D., Sherman, G., Shannon, W., & Kollef, M. (1999). Effect of a nursing-implemented sedation protocol on the duration of mechanical ventilation. *Critical Care Medicine, 27*(12), 2609–2615.

Brook, A., Sherman, G., Malen, J., & Kollef, M. (2000). Early versus late tracheostomy in patients who require prolonged mechanical ventilation. *American Journal of Critical Care, 9*(5), 352–359.

Burns, S., Marchall, M., Burns, J., Ryan, B., Wilmoth, D., Carpenter, R., Aloi, A., Wood, M., & Truwit, J. (1998). Design, testing, and results of an outcome-managed approach to patients requiring prolonged mechanical ventilation. *American Journal of Critical Care, 7*(1), 45–57.

Jardine, E., O'Toole, M., Paton, J. Y., & Wallis, C. (1999). Current status of long-term ventilation of children in the United Kingdom: Questionnaire survey. *British Medical Journal, 318*(7179), 295–299.

Leger, P. (1994). Noninvasive positive pressure ventilation at home. *Respiratory Care, 39*(5), 501–510.

Ross, B., Barker, D., Russell, W., & Burns R. (1996). Prediction of long-term ventilatory support in trauma patients. *American Surgeon, 62*(1), 19–25.

Tracheostomy Tubes

Deutsch, E. (1998). Early tracheostomy tube change in children. *Archives of Otolaryngology—Head and Neck Surgery, 124*(11), 1237–1238.

Irving, R., Jones, N., Bailey, C., & Melville, J. (1991). A guide to the selection of pediatric tracheostomy tubes. *Journal of Laryngology and Otology, 105*(12), 1046–1051.

Marlow, F., Tomkin, E., & Zwillenberg, S. (1991). Custom made tracheostomy tubes. *Ear, Nose and Throat Journal, 70*(5), 309–310.

Richardson, J., & Smith, P. (1988). Replacement of tracheostomy tubes. *Anesthesia, 43*(6), 519.

Wee, M. (1988). A speaking adaptor for a tracheostomy tube. *British Journal of Anesthesia, 61*(4), 516.

Weilitz, P., & Dettenmeier, P. (1994). Test your knowledge of tracheostomy tubes. *American Journal of Nursing, 94*(2), 46–50.

Widman, W. (1974). Technique for changing tracheostomy tubes in the early postoperative patient. *Critical Care Medicine, 2*(5), 277–278.

Wyatt, M., Bailey, C., & Whiteside, J. (1999). Update on pediatric tracheostomy tubes. *Journal of Laryngology and Otology, 113*(1), 35–40.

Discharge Planning and Homecare

Barnes, L., (1992). Tracheostomy care: Preparing parents for discharge. *Maternal-Child Nursing Journal, 17*, 293.

Baumgardner, D., & Burtea, E. (1998). Quality-of-life in technology-dependent children receiving home care, and their families—A qualitative study. *Wisconsin Medical Journal, 97*(8), 51–55.

Buzz-Kelly, L., & Gordin, P. (1993). Teaching CPR to parents of children with tracheostomies. *Maternal-Child Nursing Journal, 18*, 158–163.

Dougherty, J., Parrish, J., & Hock-Long, L. (1995). Developing a competency-based curriculum for tracheostomy and ventilator care. *Pediatric Nursing, 21*(6), 581–584.

Duncan, B., Howell, L., deLorimier, A., Adzick, N., & Harrison, M. (1992). Tracheostomy in children with emphasis on home care. *Journal of Pediatric Surgery, 27*(4), 432–435.

Fauroux, B., Sardet, A., & Foret, D. (1995). Home treatment for chronic respiratory failure in children: A prospective study. *European Respiratory Journal, 8*(12), 2062–2066.

Fitton, C. (1994). Nursing management of the child with a tracheotomy. *Pediatric Clinics of North America, 41*(3), 513–523.

Goldstein, R., Psek, J., & Gort, E. (1995). Home mechanical ventilation. Demographics and user perspectives. *Chest, 108*(6), 1581–1586.

Kenelly, C. (1987). Tracheostomy care: Parents as learners. *Maternal-Child Nursing Journal, 12*, 264–267.

Lichtenstein, M. (1986). Pediatric home tracheostomy care: A parents' guide. *Pediatric Nursing, 12*, 41–69.

Rueben, R., Newton, L., Jornsay, D., Stein, R., Chambers, H., Liquori, J., & Lawrence, C. (1982). Home care of the pediatric patient with a tracheotomy. *Annals of Otology, Rhinology and Laryngology, 91*, 633–640.

Talabere, L. (1980). The child with a tracheostomy: A holistic approach to home care. *Topics in Clinical Nursing, 2*, 27–44.

INTERNET SITES

University of Wisconsin Children's Hospital
http://www.pediatrics.wisc.edu/childrenshosp/trach/cat.html
Target Audience: Appropriate references for parents and speech language pathologists.
Content: Contains categorical bibliography with brief summaries of articles.

Aaron's Tracheostomy Page
http://www.twinenterprises.com/trach/
Target Audience: Contains information about tracheostomies that would be useful for parents and speech language pathologists.
Content: Contains information on numerous (24) topics related to tracheostomy, such as speech, feeding, a respiratory dictionary etc. This Web site also includes a chat room and a "What's new?" feature.

University of Chicago Children's Hospital
http://www.ucch.org/ucch/healthpages/pulcrit/breath/noframe/index.html
Target Audience: Contains information that would be very useful for parents.
Content: Contains basic information about tracheostomies and their care, daily management, homecare, and emergency care. This Web site includes diagrams alongside text. Information on this Web site is also available as a booklet.

University of California-Davis
http://wellness.ucdavis.edu/child_health/special_needs/pediatric_tracheostomy/
Target Audience: Contains information that would be very useful for parents.
Content: Provides specific instructions for topics such as suctioning, cleaning, and changing tracheostomy tubes, trach skin care, etc.

Passy-Muir, Inc.
http://www.passy-muir.com
Target Audience: Contains technical information about tracheostomy, tracheostomy tubes, and speaking valves appropriate for use by speech language pathologists.
Content: Contains detailed information about speaking valves and adaptors, preplacement assessment guidelines, and product descriptions.

REFERENCES

Adamson, L. B., & Dunbar, B. (1991). Communication development of young children with tracheostomies. *Augmentative and Alternative Communication, 7*, 275–283.

Albamonte, S., Jerome, A., Diwadkar, V., & Seid, A. (1993). Pediatrics. In M. F. Mason (Ed.), *Speech pathology for tracheostomized and ventilator-dependent patients.* (1st ed. pp. 383–419). Newport Beach, CA: Voicing! Inc.

Als, H. (1986). A synactive model of neonatal behavioral organization. *Physical and Occupational Therapy in Pediatrics, 6*(3/4), 3–55.

Als, H. (1997). Earliest intervention for preterm infants in the newborn intensive care unit. In M. J. Guralnick (Ed.), *The effectiveness of early intervention.* (pp. 47–76). Baltimore, MD: Paul H. Brookes Publishing Co.

Als, H., Lawhon, G., Brown, E., Gibes, R., Duffy, F., McAnulty, G., & Bickman, J. (1986). Individualized behavioral and environmental care for the very low birth weight preterm infant at high risk for bronchopulmonary dysplasia: Neonatal intensive care unit and developmental outcome. *Pediatrics, 78*, 1123–1132.

Als, H., Lawhon, G., Duffy, F., McAnulty, G., Gibes-Grossman, R., & Bickman, J. (1994). Individualized developmental care for the very low birth weight preterm infant. Medical and neurofunctional effects. *Journal of the American Medical Association, 272*, 853–858.

Als, H., Lester, B., Tronick, E. Z., & Brazelton, T. B. (1982). Toward a research instrument for the assessment of preterm infant's behavior. In H. E. Fitzgerald, B. M. Lester, & M. W. Yogman (Eds.), *Theory and research in behavioral pediatrics. Vol. 1.* (pp. 36–63). New York: Plenum Press.

American Speech-Language-Hearing Association (1989). Assessing infants and toddlers: A family focus. Videoconference. May 19, 1989.

American Speech-Language-Hearing Association (1993). Position statement and guidelines for the use of voice prosthesis in tracheostomized person with and without ventilatory dependence. *American Speech-Language-Hearing Association, 35*(Supplement 10), 17–20.

Arcand, P., & Granger, J. (1988). Pediatric tracheostomies: Changing trends. *The Journal of Otolaryngology, 17*(2), 121–124.

Arvedson, J. (1993). Oral-motor feeding assessment. In J. Arvedson and L. Brodsky (Eds.), *Pediatric swallowing and feeding: Assessment and management.* (pp. 249–292). San Diego, CA: Singular Publishing Group, Inc.

Arvedson, J. C., & Brodsky, L. (1992). Pediatric tracheotomy referrals to speech-language pathology in a children's hospital. *International Journal of Pediatric Otorhinolaryngology, 23*, 237–243.

Arvedson, J. C., & Brodsky, L. (1993). *Pediatric swallowing and feeding: Assessment and management.* San Diego, CA: Singular Publishing Group, Inc.

Bain, B., & Dollaghan, C. (1991). Clinical forum treatment efficacy: The notion of clinically significant change. *Language, Speech and Hearing Services in Schools, 22*, 264–270.

Barnes, L., (1992). Tracheostomy care: Preparing parents for discharge. *Maternal-Child Nursing Journal, 17*, 293.

Bates, E., Camaioni, L., & Volterra, V. (1975). The acquisition of performatives prior to speech. *Merrill-Palmer Quarterly, 21*, 205–224.

Bates, E., Thal, D., Whitesell, K., Fenson, L., & Oakes, L. (1989). Integrating language and gesture in infancy. *Developmental Psychology, 25*(6), 1004–1019.

Bauman-Waengler, J. (2000). *Articulatory and phonological impairments: A clinical focus.* Boston, MA: Allyn and Bacon.

Bennett, F., Silver, G., Leung, E., & Mack, L. (1990). Periventricular echo densities detected by cranial ultrasound: Usefulness in predicting neurodevelopmental outcomes in low birth weight, preterm infants. *Pediatrics, 85*, 400–404.

Billeaud, F. P. (1998). *Communication disorders in infants and toddlers: Assessment and intervention. 2nd ed.* Boston, MA: Butterworth-Heinemann.

Blache, S. (1989). A distinctive feature approach. In N. Creaghead, P. Newman, & W. Secord (Eds.), *Assessment and remediation of articulatory and phonological disorders* (*2nd ed.*, pp. 361–382). New York: Macmillan.

Bleile, K. M. (1993). *The care of children with long-term tracheostomies.* San Diego, CA: Singular Publishing Group.

Bleile, K. M. (1998). Where words come from: The origins of expressive language. In R. Paul (Ed.), *Exploring the speech-language connection. Communication and language series. Vol. 8.* (pp. 119–138). Baltimore, MD: Paul H. Brookes Publishing Co.

Bleile, K. M., & Miller, S.A. (1994). Toddlers with medical needs. In J. E. Bernthal & N. W. Bankson (Eds.), *Child phonology: Characteristics, assessment, and interventions with special populations.* (pp. 81–109). New York: Thieme Medical Publishers, Inc.

Bleile, K., Stark, R., & Silverman-McGowan, J. (1993). Speech development in a child after decannulation: Further evidence that babbling facilitates later speech development. *Clinical Linguistics and Phonetics, 7*, 319–337.

Braun, M. A., & Palmer, M. M. (1986). A pilot study of oral-motor dysfunction in "at risk" infants. *Physical and Occupational Therapy in Pediatrics, 5*(4), 13–25.

Brazelton, R. B. (1984). *Neonatal behavioral assessment scale. 2nd ed.* London: Spastics International Medical Publications.

Bricker, D. (1993) *Assessment, evaluation and programming system (AEPS) for infants and children. Vol 1. AEPS measurement for birth to three years.* Baltimore, MD: Paul H. Brookes Publishing Co.

Bricker, D., Squires, J., & Mounts, L. (1995). *Ages and stages questionnaires (ASQ): A parent-completed child-mentoring system.* Baltimore, MD: Paul H. Brookes Publishing Co.

Brodsky, L. (1997). Dysphagia with respiratory/pulmonary presentation: Assessment and management. *Seminars in Speech and Language, 18*(1), 13–23.

Bzoch, K., & League, R. (1991). *The receptive expressive language scale.* Gainesville, FL: Language Education Division, Computer Management Corporation.

Camp, B., Burgess, D., Morgan, L., & Zerbe, G. (1987). A longitudinal study of infant vocalizations in the first year. *Journal of Pediatric Psychology, 12*(3), 321–331.

Camp, B., Morgan, L., & Schmidt, B. (1987). Infant vocalization: An index of maternal attitude toward the child. *Journal of Pediatric Psychology, 12*(3), 333–341.

Case-Smith, J. (1986). An efficacy study of occupational therapy with high-risk neonates. *The American Journal of Occupational Therapy, 42*, 499–506.

Case-Smith, J., Cooper, P., & Scala, V. (1989). Feeding efficiency of premature neonates. *Journal of Occupational Therapy, 43*(4), 245–250.

Chaikind, S., & Corman, H. (1991). The impact of low birth weight on special education costs. *Journal of Health Economics, 10*(3), 291–311.

Clarke-Stewart, K. (1973). Interactions between mothers and their young children: Characteristics and consequences. *Monographs of the Society for Research in Child Development, 38*, 6–7.

Colbert, A., & Curran, F. (1991). Rehabilitation concerns in late-stage, ventilator-dependent muscular dystrophy patients. In L. I. Charach (Ed.), *Muscular dystrophy and other neuromuscular diseases: Psychological issues.* New York: Haworth Press.

Creger, P. J. (1989). *Developmental interventions for preterm and high-risk infants: Self-study modules for professionals.* Tucson, AZ: Therapy Skill Builders.

Davis, B., & MacNeilage, P. E. (1990). Acquisition of correct vowel production: A quantitative case study. *Journal of Speech and Hearing Research, 33*, 16–27.

Dikeman, K. J., & Kazandijan, M. A. (1995). Oral communication options. In K. Dikeman & M. Kazandijan (Eds.), *Communication and swallowing management of tracheostomized and ventilator-dependent adults.* (pp. 173–179). San Diego, CA: Singular Publishing Group.

Dormans, J. P., & Pellegrino, L. (1998). *Caring for children with cerebral palsy: A team approach.* Baltimore, MD: Paul H. Brookes Publishing Co.

Driver, L.E. (2000). Pediatric considerations. In D. Tippet (Ed.), *Tracheostomy and ventilator dependency: Management of breathing, speaking and swallowing.* (pp. 193–235). New York: Thieme Medical Publishers, Inc.

Duncan, B. W., Howell, L. J., deLorimier, A. A., Adzick, N. S., & Harrison, M. R. (1992). Tracheostomy in children with emphasis on home care. *Journal of Pediatric Surgery, 27*(4), 432–435.

Dunn, S., van Kleeck, A., & Rossetti, L. (1993a). Current roles and continuing needs of speech-language pathologists working in NICUs. *American Journal of Speech-Language Pathology, 2*(2), 52–64.

Dunn, S., van Kleeck, A., & Rossetti, L. (1993b). Clinical recommendations for assessment and treatment from speech-language pathologists working in neonatal intensive care units. *Infant-Toddler Intervention, 3*(4), 245–254.

Dunst, C. (1980). *A clinical and educational manual for use with the Uzgiris and Hunt scales of infant psychological development.* Austin, TX: Pro-Ed.

Fenson, L., Dale, P. S., Reznick, J. S., Thal, D., Bates, E., Hartung, J. P., Pethick, S., & Reilly, J. S. (1996). *MacArthur communicative development inventories: Words and gestures: User's guide and technical manual.* San Diego, CA: Singular Publishing Group.

Fields, A., Coble, D., Pollack, M., & Kaufman, J. (1991). Outcome of home care for technology-dependent children: Success of an independent, community-based case management model. *Pediatric Pulmonology, 11*(4), 310–317.

Fitzgerald, H. E., Lester, B. M., & Yogman, M. W. (1982). *Theory and research in behavioral pediatrics. Vol. 1.* (pp. 64–133). New York: Plenum Press.

Fleischer, B. F., VandenBerg, K. A., Constantinou, J., Heller, C., Benitz, W. E., Johnson, A., Rosenthal, A., & Stevenson, D. K. (1995). Individualized developmental care for very-low-birth weight premature infants. *Clinical Pediatrics, 34,* 523–529.

Frattali, C. M. (1998). *Measuring outcomes in speech-language pathology.* New York: Thieme Medical Publishers, Inc.

Furuno, S., O'Reilly, A., Husaka, C. M., Inatsuka, T. T., Allmon, T. L., & Zeisloft-Falbey, B. (1994). *The Hawaii early learning profile.* Palo Alto, CA: Vort Corporation.

Fus, L. A., & Wacker, D. P. (1993). The role of vocalizations on social behaviors of a tracheostomized toddler. *Infant-Toddler Intervention: The Transdisciplinary Journal, 3*(4), 237–244.

Gallagher, T., & Watkin, K. (1998). Pre-maturity and language developmental risk: Too young or too small? *Topics in Language Disorders, 18*(3), 15–25.

Gee, R., & Meredith, S. (1987). *Entertaining and educating your preschool child.* London: Usborne Publishing, Ltd.

Girolametto, L., & Ushycky, I. (1989). You and your baby: Building communication. Toronto, ON: Hanen Early Language Program.

Glass, R. B., & Wolf, L. S. (1994). A global perspective on feeding assessment in the neonatal intensive care unit. *The American Journal of Occupational Therapy, 48*(6), 514–526.

Goldberg, S. (1977). Social competence in infancy: A model of parent-infant interaction. *Merrill-Palmer Quarterly, 23,* 163–177.

Goldson, E. (1996). The micropremie: Infants with birth weight less than 800 grams. *Infants and Young Children, 8*(3), 1–10.

Handler, S. D. (1993). Surgical management of the tracheostomy. In K. M. Bleile (Ed.), *The care of children with long-term tracheostomy.* (pp. 33–40). San Diego, CA: Singular Publishing Group, Inc.

Harris, M. (1986). Oral-motor management of the high-risk neonate. *Physical and Occupational Therapy in Pediatrics, 6*(3), 231–253.

Hill, B. P., & Singer, L. T. (1990). Speech and language development after infant tracheostomy. *Journal of Speech and Hearing Research, 55,* 15–20.

Hodson, B. W. (1986). *The assessment of phonological processes—revised.* Danville, IL: Interstate.

Hodson, B. W., & Paden, E. P. (1991). *Targeting intelligible speech: A phonological approach to remediation. 2nd ed.* San Diego, CA: College Hill Press.

Iverson, J. M., & Thal, D. J. (1998). Communicative transitions: There's more to the hand than meets the eye. In A. Wetherby, S. Warren, & J. Reichle (Eds.), *Transitions in prelinguistic communication. Vol. 7.* (pp. 59–86). Baltimore, MD: Paul H. Brookes Publishing Co.

Johnson-Martin, N. M., Jens, K. G., Attermeier, S. M., & Hacker, B. J. (1991). *The Carolina curriculum for infants and toddlers with special needs. 2nd ed. Manual.* Baltimore, MD: Paul H. Brookes Publishing Co.

Kamen, R. S., & Watson, B. C. (1991). Effects of long-term tracheostomy on spectral characteristics of vowel production. *Journal of Speech and Hearing Research, 34,* 1057–1065.

Kaslon, K. W., & Stein, R. E. (1985). Chronic pediatric tracheostomy: Assessment and implications for habilitation of voice, speech and language in young children. *International Journal of Pediatric Otorhinolaryngology, 9*, 165–171.

Katz, K., Pokorni, J., & Long, T. (1989). *Chronologically ill and at risk infants: Family centered intervention from hospital to home.* Palo Alto, CA: Vort Corporation.

Kaufman, A., & Kaufman, N. (1983). *Kaufman assessment battery for children.* Circle Pines, MN: American Guidance Service.

Kennedy, A. H., Johnson, N. G., & Sturdevant, E. W. (1982). An educational program for families of children with tracheostomies. *American Journal of Maternal-Child Nursing*, 42–49.

Kenny, D., Koheil, R., Greenberg, J., Reid, D., Milner, M., Roman, R., & Judd, P. (1989). Development of a multidisciplinary feeding profile for children who are dependent feeders. *Dysphagia, 4*, 16–28.

Kent, R.D. (1998). Normal aspects of articulation. In J. E. Bernthal & N. W. Bankson (Eds.), *Articulation and phonological disorders. 4th ed.* (pp. 1–62). Boston, MA: Allyn & Bacon.

Kersten, L. D. (1989). Tracheostomy and tracheostomy tubes. In L. D. Kersten (Ed.), *Comprehensive respiratory nursing: A decision making approach.* (pp. 652–699). Toronto, ON: W. B. Saunders Co.

Kertoy, M. K., Guest, C. M., Quart, E., & Lieh-Lai, M. (1999). Speech and phonological characteristics of individual children with a history of tracheostomy. *Journal of Speech, Language, and Hearing Research, 42*(3), 621–635.

Kertoy, M. K., & Morrison, A. A. (2000). Gesture use by two children with tracheostomy: Getting ready to use words. In M. Perkins & S. Howard (Eds.), *New directions in language development and disorders.* (pp. 61–72). New York: Plenum Publishers.

Kertoy, M. K., & Waters, R. (1995). Communicative intentions of three prelinguistic children with a history of long-term tracheostomy. *Infant-Toddler Intervention, 5*(3), 301–314.

Kleinsasser, N., Merkenschlager, A., Schroter, C., Mattick, C., Nicolai, T., & Mantel, K. (1996). Fatal complications in tracheotomized children. *Laryngorhinootologie, 75*(2), 77–82.

Kuhl, P., & Meltzoff, A. (1982). The bimodal perception of speech in infancy. *Science, 218*, 1138–1141.

Laadt-Bruno, G., Lilley, P. K., & Westby, C. E. (1993). A collaborative approach to developmental care continuity with infants born at risk and their families. *Topics in Language Disorders, 14*(1), 15–28.

Lehman, J. A., Fishman, J. R., & Neiman, G. S. (1995). Treatment of cleft palate associated with Pierre Robin sequence: Appraisal of risk factors. *Cleft Palate and Craniofacial Journal, 32*(1), 25–29.

Levitt, C., Watters, N., Chance, G., Walker, R., & Avard, D. (1993). Low-birth-weight symposium: Summary of proceedings. *Canadian Medical Association Journal, 148*(5), 767–772.

Lieberman, P. (1980). On the development of vowel production in young children. In G. H. Yeni-Komshian, J. F. Kavanaugh, & C. A. Ferguson (Eds.), *Child phonology. Vol. 1.* (pp. 23–42). New York: Academic Press.

Linder, T. (1993). *Transdisciplinary play-based assessment: A functional approach to working with young children.* Baltimore, MD: Paul H. Brookes Publishing Co.

Locke, J. L. (1987). Are developmental language disorders primarily grammatical? Paper presented at the Child Language Seminar, Department of Human Communication Sciences, University of Sheffield, Sheffield, UK, Sept. 1998.

Locke, J. L., & Pearson, D. M. (1990). Linguistic significance of babbling: Evidence from a tracheostomized infant. *Journal of Child Language, 17*, 1–6.

Locke, J. F., & Pearson, D. M. (1992). Vocal learning and the emergence of phonological capacity: A neurological approach. In C. A. Ferguson, L. Menn, & C. Stoel-Gammon (Eds.), *Phonological development: Models, research, implications.* (pp. 91–130). Timonium, MD: York Press, Inc.

Logemann, J. A. (2000). What is evidence-based practice and why should we care? *The ASHA Leader, 5*(5), 3.

Lowe, M., & Costello, A. (1988). *Symbolic play test. 2nd ed.* Austin, TX: Pro-Ed.

MacWhinney, B. (1989). *Child language analysis. Manual for use of the CLAN programs for the child language data exchange.* Pittsburgh, PA: Dept. of Psychology, Carnegie Mellon University.

Manley, S. B., Frank, E. M., & Melvin, C. F. (1999). Preparation of speech-language pathologists to provide services to patients with a tracheostomy tube: A survey. *American Journal of Speech-Language Pathology, 8*(2), 172–180.

Manolson, A. (1992). *It takes two to talk: A parent's guide to helping children communicate.* Toronto, ON: The Hanen Center.

Martin, B., & Carle, E. (1995). *Brown bear, brown bear, what do you see?* New York: Henry Holt & Co.

Mason, M. F. (1993). *Speech pathology for tracheostomized and ventilator-dependent patients. 1st ed.* Newport Beach, CA: Voicing! Inc.

Mason, M., & Watkins, C. (1992). Communication for the tracheostomized and ventilator patient utilizing the Passy-Muir valve. Paper presented at Technology and Persons with Disabilities Conference. California State University, Northridge, California, March 18–21, 1992.

McCune, L. (1995). A normative study of representational play at the transition to language. *Developmental Psychology, 31*, 200–211.

McReynolds, L. V., & Kearns, K. P. (1983). *Single-subject experimental designs in communicative disorders.* Baltimore, MD: University Park Press.

Meisels, S., Jones, S., & Steifel, G. (1983). Neonatal intervention: Problem, purpose, and prospects. *Topics in Early Childhood Special Education, 3*(1), 1–13.

Meisels, S. J., Plunkett, J. W., Pasick, P. L., Steifel, G. S., & Roloff, D. W. (1987). Effects or severity and chronicity of respiratory illness on the cognitive development of preterm infants. *Journal of Pediatric Psychology, 12*(1), 117–132.

Meltzoff, A. N. (1986). Imitation, intermodal representation, and the origins of mind. In B. Lindblom & T. Zetterstrom (Eds.), *Precursors of early speech.* New York: Stockton Press.

Miller, J. (1981). *Assessing language production in children: Experimental procedures.* Needham Heights, MA: Allyn and Bacon.

Miller, M., & Quinn-Hurst, M. (1994). Neurobehavioral assessment of high-risk infants in the neonatal intensive care unit. *The American Journal of Occupational Therapy, 48*(6), 506–513.

Morris, S.E. (1981). *The normal acquisition of oral feeding skills: Implications for assessment and treatment.* Workshop proceedings, Boston, MA: June 20–23.

Morris, S. E., & Klein, M. D. (1987). *Pre-feeding skills: A comprehensive resource for feeding development.* Tucson, AZ: Therapy Skill Builders.

Morrison, A. A. (1998). An investigation of communication behaviors in prelinguistic tracheostomized children. Unpublished Master's Thesis, University of Western Ontario, London, Ontario, September, 1998.

Nelson, M. N. (1993). Indices of disordered development. Paper presented at the symposium, High-risk infants: Individualized care and developmental support for the high-risk and preterm infant from the NICU to home and school-based programs. Henry Ford Hospital, Warren, Michigan, June 8–9, 1993.

Norris, J. A., & Hoffman, P. R. (1990). Comparison of adult initiated vs. child initiated interaction styles with handicapped prelanguage children. *Language, Speech and Hearing Services in Schools, 21*(1), 28–36

Office of Technology Assessment (1987). *Technology dependent children: Hospital vs. home care—A technical memorandum.* Washington, DC. Author.

Oller, D. K., & Eilers, R. E. (1988). The role of audition in infant babbling. *Child Development, 59*, 444–449.

Olswang, L. B. (1998). Treatment efficacy research. In C. M. Frattali (Ed.), *Measuring outcomes in speech-language pathology.* (pp. 134–150). New York: Thieme Medical Publishers, Inc.

Olswang, L., & Pinder, G. L. (1995). Preverbal functional communication and the role of object play in children with cerebral palsy. *Infant-Toddler Intervention: The Transdisciplinary Journal, 5*(3), 277–300.

Olswang, L., Stoel-Gammon, C., Coggins, T., & Carpenter, R. (1987). *Assessing linguistic behaviors.* Seattle, WA: University of Washington Press.

Owens, R. (1996). *Language development: An introduction. 4th ed.* New York: Macmillan.

Owens, R. (1999). *Language disorders: A functional approach to assessment and intervention. 3rd ed.* Needham Heights, MA: Allyn & Bacon.

Parker, S. J., Zahr, L. K., Cole, J. G., & Brecht, M. (1992). Outcome after developmental intervention in the neonatal intensive care unit for mothers of preterm infants with low socioeconomic status. *Journal of Pediatrics, 120*, 78–785.

Paul, R. (1995). *Language disorders from infancy through adolescence: Assessment and intervention.* St. Louis, MO: Mosby.

Paul, R., & Jennings, P. (1992). Phonological behavior in toddlers with slow expressive language development. *Journal of Speech and Hearing Research, 35*, 99–107.

Pinder, G. L., & Olswang, L. (1995). Development of communicative intent in young children with cerebral palsy: A treatment efficacy study. *Infant-Toddler Intervention: The Transdisciplinary Journal, 5*(1), 51–70.

Pinelli, J., & Symington, A. (2000). How rewarding can a pacifier be? A systematic review of nonnutritive sucking in preterm infants. *Neonatal Network, 19*(8), 41–48.

Pollack, K. E. (1991). The identification of vowel errors using traditional articulation or phonological process test stimuli. *Language, Speech and Hearing Services in Schools, 22*, 39–50.

Preisser, D., Hodson, B., & Paden, E. (1988). Developmental phonology: 18–29 months. *Journal of Speech and Hearing Disorders, 53*, 125–130.

Proctor, A. (1989). Stages of normal non-cry vocal development in infancy: A protocol for assessment. *Topics in Language Disorders, 10*(1), 26–42.

Prodoehl, D. C., & Shuttuck, K. E. (1995). Nasogastric intubation for nutrition and airway protection in infants with Pierre Robin sequence. *Journal of Perinatology, 15*(5), 395–397.

Rathlev, M. C., & McNamara, M. A. (1982). Teaching families to give trach care at home. *Nursing, 11*(6), 81–82.

Richardson, M., Student, E., O'Boyle, D., Smyth, M., & Wheeler, T. W. (1992). Establishment of a state-supported, specialized home care program for children with complex health care needs. *Issues in Comprehensive Pediatric Nursing, 15*(2), 93–122.

Rogers, B. T. (1996). Neurodevelopmental presentation of dysphagia. *Seminars in Speech and Language, 17*(4), 269–281.

Ross, G. S. (1982). Language functioning and speech development of six children receiving tracheotomy in infancy. *Journal of Communication Disorders, 15*, 95–111.

Rossetti, L. M. (1990). *The Rossetti infant-toddler language scale: A measure of communication and interaction.* East Moline, IL: LinguiSystems.

Rossetti, L. M. (2001). *Communication intervention. Birth to three. 2nd ed.* Albany, NY: Singular/Thomson Learning.

Secord, W. (1985). The traditional approach to articulation treatment. In P. Newman, N. Creaghead, & W. Secord (Eds.), *Assessment and remediation of articulation and phonological disorders.* (pp. 127–158). Columbus, OH: Merrill Publishing.

Seuss, Dr. (1960). *Green eggs and ham.* New York: Random House.

Sheppard, J. J. (1987). Assessment of oral motor behaviours in cerebral palsy. *Seminars in Speech and Language, 8*(1), 57–69.

Shinkwin, C. A., & Gibbin, K. P. (1996). Tracheostomy in children. *Journal of the Royal Society of Medicine, 4*, 188–192.

Silverman-McGowan, J., Bleile, K. M., Fus, L., & Barnas, E. (1993). Communication disorders. In K. M. Bleile (Ed.), *The care of children with long-term tracheostomies.* (pp. 113–140). San Diego, CA: Singular Publishing Group.

Simon, B., & Handler, S. (1981). The speech pathologist and management of children with tracheostomies. *Journal of Otolaryngology, 10*, 440–448.

Simon, B. M., Fowler, S. M., & Handler, S. D. (1983). Communication development in young children with long-term tracheostomies: Preliminary report. *International Journal of Pediatric Otorhinolaryngology, 6*, 37–60.

Singer, L. T., Kercsmar, C., Legris, G., Orlowski, J. P., Hill, B. J., & Doershuck, C. (1989). Developmental sequelae of long-term tracheostomy. *Developmental Medicine and Child Neurology, 31*, 224–230.

Singer, L. T., Wood, R., & Lambert, S. (1985). Developmental follow-up of long-term infant tracheostomy: A preliminary report. *Developmental and Behavioral Pediatrics, 6*(3), 132–136.

Slonim, A. D., Patel, K. M., Ruttiman, U. E., & Pollack, M. M. (2000). *Critical Care Medicine, 28*(3), 848–853.

Snow, C. E. (1989). Initiativeness: A trait or a skill? In G. E. Speidel & K. E. Nelson (Eds.), *The many faces of imitation in language learning.* New York: Springer-Verlag.

Sparrow, S., Balla, D., & Cicchetti, D. (1984). *Vineland adaptive behavior scales.* Circle Pines, MN: American Guidance Service.

Stoel-Gammon, C. (1985). Phonetic inventories 15–24 months: A longitudinal study. *Journal of Speech and Hearing Research, 28*, 505–512.

Stoel-Gammon, C. (1992). Prelinguistic vocal development: Measurement and predictions. In C. A. Ferguson, L. Menn, & C. Stoel-Gammon (Eds.), *Phonological development: Models, research, implications.* (pp. 439–456). Timonium, MD: York Press.

Stoel-Gammon, C., & Herrington, P. (1990). Vowel systems of normally developing and phonologically disordered children. *Clinical Linguistics and Phonetics, 4*, 145–160.

Stoel-Gammon, C., & Otomo, K. (1986). Babbling development of hearing impaired and normally hearing subjects. *Journal of Speech and Hearing Disorders, 51*, 33–41.

Tannock, R., & Girolametto, L. (1992). Reassessing parent-focused language intervention programs. In S. F. Warren & J. Reichle (Eds.), *Communication and language intervention series. Vol. 1. Causes and effects in communication and language intervention.* (pp. 49–79). Baltimore, MD: Paul H. Brookes Publishing Co.

Thal, D., & Bates, E. (1988). Language and gesture in late talkers. *Journal of Speech and Hearing Research, 31*, 115–123.

Thal, D., & Tobias, S. (1994). Relationships between language and gesture in normally developing and late-talking toddlers. *Journal of Speech and Hearing Research, 37*(1), 157–170.

Thal, D., Tobias, S., & Morrison, D. (1991). Language and gesture in late talkers: A 1-year follow-up. *Journal of Speech and Hearing Research, 34*, 604–612.

Tippet, D. (2000). *Tracheostomy and ventilator dependency: Management of breathing, speaking and swallowing.* New York: Thieme Medical Publishers, Inc.

VandenBerg, K. A. (1993). Basic competencies to begin developmental care in the intensive care nursery. *Infants and Young Children, 6*(2), 52–59.

VandenBerg, K. A. (1999). What to tell parents about the developmental needs of their baby at discharge. *Neonatal Network, 18*(1), 57–59.

VandenBerg, K. A., & Franck, L. S. (1990). Behavioral issues for infants with BPD. In C. Lund (Ed.), *Bronchopulmonary dysplasia—Building strategies for total patient care.* (pp. 113–152). Petaluma: *Neonatal Network.*

Velleman, S. L., & Strand, K. E. (1998). Dynamic remediation strategies for children with developmental verbal apraxia. Videotape and Manual. Rockville, MD: American Speech and Hearing Association.

Vihman, M. M. (1992). Early syllables and the construction of phonology. In C. A. Ferguson, L. Menn, & C. Stoel-Gammon (Eds.), *Phonological development: Models, research, implications.* (pp. 393–422). Timonium, MD: York Press.

Vihman, M. M., & Greenlee, M. (1987). Individual differences in phonological development: Ages one and three years. *Journal of Speech and Hearing Research, 30*, 503–521.

Warren, S. F., & Yoder, P. J. (1998). Facilitating the transition from preintentional to intentional communication. In A. Wetherby, S. Warren, & J. Reichle (Eds.), *Transitions in prelinguistic communication* (*Vol. 7*. pp. 365–384). Baltimore, MD: Paul H. Brookes Publishing Co.

Weitzman, E. (1992). *Learning language and loving it. A guide to promoting children's social and language development in early childhood settings.* (pp. 49–55). Toronto, ON: The Hanen Center.

Wetherby, A., Cain, D., Yonclas, D., & Walker, V. (1988). Analysis of intentional communication of normal children from the prelinguistic to the multi-word stage. *Journal of Speech and Hearing Research, 31*, 240–252.

Wetherby, A., & Prizant, B. (1993). *Communication and symbolic behavior scales. 1st ed.* Chicago, IL: Riverside Publishing.

Wetherby, A., & Prutting, C. (1984). Profiles of communicative and cognitive-social abilities in autistic children. *Journal of Speech and Hearing Research, 27*, 364–377.

Wetherby, A., Yonclas, D., & Bryan, A. (1989). Communication profiles of preschool children with handicaps: Implications for early identification. *Journal of Speech and Hearing Disorders, 54*, 148–158.

Wetmore, R. F., Marsh, R., Thompson, M. E., & Tom, L. W. (1999). Pediatric tracheostomy: A changing procedure? *Annals of Otology, Rhinology & Laryngology, 108*(7), 695–699.

Willis, J. M. (1983). Concerns and needs of mothers providing home care for children with tracheostomies. *Maternal-Child Nursing Journal, 12*(2), 89–107.

Wyly, M., Allen, J., Pfalzer, S., & Wilson, J. (1996). Providing a seamless service system from hospital to home: The NICU Training Project. *Infants and Young Children, 8*(3), 77–84.

Yoder, P. J. (1987). Relationship between degree of infant handicap and clarity of infant cues. *American Journal of Mental Deficiency, 91*(6), 639–641.

Yoder, P. J., & Feagans, L. (1988). Mothers' attributions of communication to prelinguistic behavior of developmentally delayed and mentally retarded infants. *American Journal on Mental Retardation, 93*(1), 36–43.

Yoder, P., Warren, S., McCarthren, R., & Leew, S. V. (1998). Does adult responsivity to child behavior facilitate communication development? In A. Wetherby, S. Warren, & J. Reichle (Eds.), *Transitions in prelinguistic communication* (*Vol. 7*. pp. 39–58). Baltimore, MD: Paul H. Brookes Publishing Co.

Zimmerman, I. L., Steiner, V., & Pond, R. E. (1992). *Preschool language scale-3.* San Antonio, TX: The Psychological Corporation.

INDEX

I

K

L

M

N

O

P

R

S

T

V